Malaria

How to Treatment and Prevention of Malaria

(The Lack of Evidence as a Significant Contributor to the High Mortality)

Norman Luna

I0089847

Published By **Regina Loviusher**

Norman Luna

All Rights Reserved

Malaria: How to Treatment and Prevention of Malaria (The Lack of Evidence as a Significant Contributor to the High Mortality)

ISBN   978-0-9959962-7-4

Legal & Disclaimer

Table Of Contents

Chapter 1: Overview Of Malaria.............. 1

Chapter 2: Malaria Vaccines 21

Chapter 3: Measures To Avoid Mosquitoes
.... 38

Chapter 4: The Malaria Vaccine For Travel
.... 45

Chapter 5: Effect Of The Malaria Vaccine
On The Global World 49

Chapter 6: Causes Of Malaria................. 57

Chapter 7: Symptoms Of Malaria 65

Chapter 8: Diagnosis Of Malaria............. 73

Chapter 9: Medications And Therapies For
Treating Malaria 79

Chapter 10: Natural And Home Remedies
For Managing Malaria Symptoms 88

Chapter 11: Preventing Malaria 96

Chapter 12: The Role Of Vaccines In
Preventing And Treating Malaria 101

Chapter 13: Combating Malaria 104

Chapter 14: The Life Cycle Of The
Mosquito 111

Chapter 15: The Mosquito 116

Chapter 16: Mosquito-Borne Encephalitis
Diseases 125

Chapter 17: Preventing Mosquito Bites 132

Chapter 18: Malaria 140

Chapter 19: Factors Which Reduce Our
Immune System 155

Chapter 20: Things You Should Know
About Malaria Attack 167

Chapter 21: Malaria 174

Chapter 22: Chikungunya 180

Chapter 1: Overview Of Malaria

Malaria is caused by the parasites that comprise the Plasmodium species. They are single-celled organic creatures with various phases of life. They require at least one host to sustain its longevity. The parasite can be transmitted to humans through mosquito bites. Patients with malaria usually suffer from severe debilitation, accompanied by shaken chill and a high fever.

Plasmodium falciparum Plasmodium Viax Plasmodium ovale Plasmodium malariae and Plasmodium knowlesi are five species of parasites that can infect human beings. The variant of Plasmodium falciparum which poses the highest threat to humans is the topic on the vast majority of research. As that the genome for P. falciparum has been successfully sequenced, scientists have improved their understanding of how they can identify the strain.

Malaria, meaning "bad air" in Italian and is the source of the word malaria. There was a belief among people that the illness was spread via miasmas, which is contaminated air before the invention of germ theory. Ronald Ross, a British doctor, found that mosquitoes were the disease's carriers. The parasite then is only carried via female Anopheles mosquitoes. Males are not able to consume blood. Females of all 60 varieties of Anopheles mosquitoes could be malaria vectors.

The disease is still common across subtropical and tropical nations despite being rare in warmer climates. Over 400,000 sufferers die every year from malaria, that's 300 million.

Malaria Transmission Cycle

Infected mosquitoes contract malaria when it bites an infected person, then biting another not infected. The malaria parasites get into the individual's circulation system before moving into the liver. The parasites attack red blood cells. They go away from the liver once they are mature.

If you eat the food of a person suffering from malaria, mosquitoes become infected.

Transmission of parasites When you bite repeatedly, it could transmit malaria parasites.

In the liver: After getting into your body, parasites migrate to your liver. There, some may become slow for up to one year.

In the bloodstream: Once they reach the maturity stage and exit the liver they invade your the red blood cells of your body. This is generally the time that symptoms of malaria begin to manifest.

On to the next. In this stage of the cycle when a mosquito doesn't have malaria bites you then it's infected by malaria parasites, and could transmit them to other people.

Since the parasites responsible for malaria infect the red blood cells, individuals may also contract malaria exposed to blood with malaria.

Other methods of transmission are:

Required by blood transfusions

Sharing drug injection needles

When the mosquito population increases

Transmission tends to be more frequent especially in areas of rurality during dry season. (though urban transmission is also seen across cities, notably in India as well as Africa).

Advice on the neighborhood malaria threat is essential to all travelers.

Symptoms of Malaria

It is sometimes difficult to distinguish malaria-related symptoms from the symptoms of influenza or other tropical illnesses like dengue diarrhoea, travelers' diarrhea or typhoid fever. In general, until confirmed that it is not, any illness that develops after traveling to an area infected with malaria must be treated as malaria. A thorough clinical examination is essential. The symptoms typically manifest one to three weeks following infection however, they can persist for up to one year following the initial exposure. The symptoms of malaria can include those listed below:

fever

chills

general discomfort

headache

nausea and vomiting

diarrhoea

Abdominal discomfort

Muscle or joint discomfort

fatigue Rapid breathing

rapid heart rate

coughs

Most often, an attack will begin by shivering and chills. It can be followed by and then an increase in temperature and sweating. It then return to normal temperatures. Malaria symptoms typically start within 10 to 30 days after the infection. Based on the type of parasite in question, the effects are not always severe. Certain people do not feel sick for up to one year following a bite from a mosquito. There is a possibility for bugs to persist in the body for several years and not cause any signs.

Based on the kind of parasite, certain types of malaria can develop a recurrence. In the course of years, when there is no activity in the liver, parasites eventually release into the bloodstream. As the parasites begin to circulate in your blood, you'll notice symptoms returning.

Causes of Malaria

A single-celled parasite from the species Plasmodium is a major cause of malaria. It is usually transmitted to humans by bites or mosquitoes. Women who are pregnant with malaria could often transmit the illness to their children who are not yet born prior to or during the birth. Congenital malaria is the term for this.

Because malaria spreads by blood, it may also be transmitted through

blood transfusions,

organ donations,

Hypodermic needles could be a vector for malaria transmission. However it is extremely unlikely.

Risk Factor of Malaria

Factors that can increase the risk to contract malaria comprise being in areas that are malaria-endemic. Subtropical and tropical areas consist of:

Sub-Saharan Africa,

South and Southeast Asia,

Pacific Islands,

Central and the northern region of South America

The risk level can be determined through measures used to protect yourself from being bitten by mosquitoes, seasonal variations in the rate of malaria, as well as the local malaria prevention.

The risk of developing more serious illnesses People who are following have a higher risk of developing grave illnesses:

Baby and small children

More experienced grown-ups

Explorers from areas with no intestinal illness

Girls and pregnant women as well as their unborn children

In many countries with significant rates of malaria The problem is made worse because of the absence of prevention measures, considerations for clinical as well as data.

Resistance can disappear

Residents of malaria-prone areas could be exposed with the illness enough to experience a slight vulnerability, which could reduce the severity of adverse consequences. A partial immune system is, however could disappear in the event that you move to an area in which you're not often exposed to the parasite.

Complications of Malaria

The disease can cause death and can be fatal, particularly if it's caused by the specific African plasmodium species. Based on the World Health Organization, approximately 94% of all deaths caused by malaria are found within Africa and most often in children who are under five years of age.

The majority of malaria-related deaths result from at the very least one of these serious issues such as:

Cerebral Malaria in the event that platelets that are contaminated with parasites block small vessels to the cerebrum (cerebral the disease of the jungle) it can cause enlargement of the mind or harm to your mind could occur. Cerebral intestinal illness can trigger seizures as well as extreme lethargies.

Problems with breathing: edema, where fluid accumulates in the lungs, may cause breathing difficulties.

Organic failure: Malaria may affect the liver and kidneys and cause the spleen rupture. All of these issues could cause a death to a patient.

Anaemia: Anaemia is the absence of blood vessels in order to provide oxygen to tissues in the body could be an indication of malaria.

Low glucose: Extreme varieties of the disease known as jungle fever may result in low glucose (hypoglycemia) in the same way as quinine, a common medication used to treat stomach sickness. The death or coma could occur due to extreme low blood sugar.

Malaria might repeat

Certain varieties of intestinal illness parasite that typically cause milder forms of infections, could last for a considerable period of time, and can cause backslides.

Prevention of Malaria

The World Health Organization distributes insecticide-treated beds nets and other preventive medication to the population to decrease the incidence of malaria-related infections. In the World Health Organization has recommended that children from countries with an elevated prevalence of malaria get an injection.

Be aware of the dangers of getting bit by a mosquito If you reside or travel to the area in which malaria is a common occurrence. Between dusk and dawn mosquitoes are the most active. It is recommended to take the following steps to prevent being bit by mosquitoes:

Hover over your skin. Dress in long-sleeved pants and shirts. Wear your shirt, and then tuck your legs of your pants in socks.

Make sure to cover your skin with repellent. If your skin is exposed, use an insect repellent approved by the Environmental Protection Agency. DEET, picaridin, IR3535, oil of lemon eucalyptus (OLE), para-menthane-3,8-diol (PMD), and 2-undecanone are examples of such repellents. Try to avoid splashing everywhere. Chemicals containing p-Menthane-3.8-diol (PMD) or oils of lemon Eucalyptus (OLE) are not to be administered to children who are under the age of three.

Apply repellent to your clothing: Sprays containing permethrin can be safely applied to clothes.

Rest in the net. The nets on your bed, specifically ones that are treated with insecticides such as permethrin can help to ward off insects while you're lying down.

Life-threatening cases of malaria are preventable by

On each journey Be aware of any areas that have malaria.

Preventing bites from mosquitoes and when required, using malaria medications

Anti malaria medication malaria is used to treat the classic and potentially deadly case of the disease. However, it is and not as an illness.

A blood test may provide the diagnosis, however several tests are possible. A number of medications used in a medical setting might be a component of the treatment. In general, local medical professionals and facilities that are practicing in areas contaminated by jungle fever have a good understanding of treating this illness. They will recommend an appropriate course of action.

There are many various kinds of medications available for the prevention of intestinal disease. It is essential to be selected by weighing the following factors:

Where to go, and what type of malaria is there.

The nature and length of the trip.

Explorer's history as a clinician.

There is no malaria medicine that can be 100% effective to stop chomps with repellent for bugs and a bed net whenever needed remains important. There's no antigen available. The local populations living in areas with malaria generally have partial immunity so they may be less susceptible to malaria than visitors.

Every malaria prescription is a winner and a hindrance. In order to help you understand what each one of them is depending on the situation, alternatives are detailed in the following.

There are risks associated with every medication. The majority of the time they're not too serious however it's recommended to be aware of the rare but potentially dangerous reactions, which should be discussed with a travel medical professional.

Preventive medicine

If you're planning to visit an area that is prone to malaria Ask your physician several months ahead of time whether you're required to take malaria-protective medicines prior to, during as well as after your travels. The medicines used for treating malaria are usually similar to those used for prevention. The exact dosage depends on the location you're traveling to, how long you're traveling for, as well as your health.

A variety of factors decide the kind of antimalarial medicine that is prescribed such as:

A person's location for travel as well as family and health history, age and even pregnancy are all aspects to be considered. Certain areas are where parasites can be resistant to specific medicines.

Doxycycline, chloroquine and a mix of proguanil and atovaquone are commonly used as preventive agents against malaria. Because certain parasites are intolerant to specific medicines, antimalarials are able to only be employed in certain regions of the globe. Since Plasmodium falciparum is totally resistant to chloroquine throughout Africa and Asia this means it cannot be treated in areas in South America with chloroquine. Prior to entering an area with a high incidence of malaria most treatment regimens for malaria must be started. This allows the medicine to be administered at the appropriate levels. Furthermore, it provides travelers with the chance to assess any potential adverse negative effects before traveling. To be able to take care of the malaria time of incubation, one must continue to take the malaria medications after returning to home.

Intermittent preventive therapy, also known as IPT can be provided to expectant mothers who reside in areas that have high or moderate malaria risk. That means they get treatment for malaria on a frequent schedule throughout the pregnancy, usually at every prenatal appointment following the 1st trimester. The presence of malaria during pregnancy is an important general medical problem. The result could be extreme malaria for the mother, premature birth, or even a baby who is born with a low weight. IPT can help approximately 32 million mothers throughout sub-Saharan African countries every year. But getting doctors to prescribe it to pregnancies ladies has proved to be a struggle. The infants who live in moderate or high-risk zones typically get the antimalarials every month along with routine medical attention during times when malaria is at an all-time high.

Treatment for Malaria

If detected early enough If caught early enough, malaria can be eliminated and managed. The issue of drug resistance, on contrary is becoming a major issue which is threatening the combat against malaria.

A majority of patients will be completely recovered if malaria is treated and diagnosed promptly. The treatment for malaria depends on many factors including:

What is the species of malaria parasite and its extent? which has triggered the illness (for example, Plasmodium falciparum)

the area of the globe where that the disease spread to

If any tablets to prevent malaria were used.

The disease can be controlled and prevented by taking medications to eliminate the parasite responsible for the illness. The medications they use are known as antimalarials. But, since malaria can be intolerant to these medications and therefore, they are not suitable to treat malaria when you are taking a specific form of antimalarial. The life cycle and biology of the parasite is affected by different drugs. Primaquine, for instance, removes dormant stages of the liver while chloroquine targets blood stage of the life cycle. To make sure that the malaria parasite gets completely eliminated from the body, drugs commonly are combined. Plasmodium Viral can be controlled by utilizing chloroquine and primaquine as an example.

Furthermore, drug combination strategies can be used to prevent parasites from developing individual resistance to drugs. Combination therapy with artemisinin (ACT) uses a method of combining the drug of one with an artemisinin-based drug, utilizes this method. ACT is currently the most advanced treatment available for malarial psoriasis. The illness can recur when parasites persist in the body following treatment. However, even if the parasites have been eliminated from the rest of the body Plasmodium vivax as well as Plasmodium ovale may remain inactive and in hiding within the liver. It is possible that the disease will return or even years after when the parasite has not been taken out of the liver correctly. Even though it does not develop to full immunity the partial immunity could decrease the severity of the illness and increase the chance of passing away from malaria over the course of. A majority of the cases of malaria from jungle fever happen for children under the age of five years old whose bodies haven't had an opportunity to build any immunity to parasites.

The relationship between sickle cell characteristic

As time passes, researchers have found that those who suffer from sickle cell disease are immune to Plasmodium falciparum, which causes malaria in one way or another. The sickle-shaped red blood cells bind to parasites, and assist in eliminating them.

Chapter 2: Malaria Vaccines

The vaccine currently developing to help prevent malaria is called the malaria vaccine. Plasmodium, which is a parasite is responsible for the ailment that is known as malaria. The disease is transmitted by mosquito bites. The issue of malaria is one of the biggest to public health, specifically in Africa's sub-Saharan region in which it kills majority of children below five years old each year, and is responsible for a large number of deaths.

The immune system is taught to detect and combat the malaria parasite prior to it causes disease. This is the manner in which the malaria vaccine functions. A protein which is located on the outside of the malaria parasite can be found in the vaccine which triggers an immune response within the body. Antibodies develop by the immune system's response. This stops the parasite from getting into red blood cells, and infecting the body through recognizing and destroying the parasite.

The development of the malaria vaccine has proved long and difficult, with many failures. However, the findings from recent studies have proven positive. The RTS,S vaccine has been found to be effective at 50% in preventing malaria among children in the early years. As part of an extensive deployment program, the vaccine is being tested across a variety of African countries.

Although the development of a malaria vaccine is an enormous step forward in fighting malaria, it's important to remember that it isn't an all-in-one solution. Lack of healthcare access as well as environmental issues such as climate change are some of the causes of the growth of malaria as well as its effects. A complete strategy that incorporates methods for controlling, treatment and prevention is essential if the disease is effectively completely eradicated.

A brief explanation of the Science of Malaria Vaccine

The vaccination's underlying science is to train the immune system to detect and eliminate malaria parasite before it causes the disease. Plasmodium an organism which infects mosquitoes, and then transmits the disease, is at the root of malaria. Chills, fever, as well as other symptoms of flu can be caused by the parasite's infecting red blood cells.

The circumsporozoite (CSP) protein can be found on the outside of malaria parasites, is the main target for the vaccine against malaria. The protein plays a role in the basic phases of intestinal illness, which occurs when the parasite is introduced into the liver, and begins increasing. The vaccine has the ability to trigger an immune response that is able to recognize the parasite, and fight it off before it is able to cause illness because it concentrates on CSP. The vaccine is comprised of a tiny bit of CSP which is called the CSP antigen. It is combined by an adjuvant that helps to strengthen the immune response. The immune system starts to create antibodies capable of recognising and attacking malaria parasites when the vaccine enters the body. The immune system recognizes CSP as a foreign CSP antigen as being foreign. This can prevent parasites from infecting the red platelets. This is the point at which symptoms become more suggestive.

To assess the safety and efficacy of this vaccine many years of study and clinical studies were carried out. The antigen has been subjected to extensive testing to confirm that it's safe and potent, as well as choose the most effective dosing regimen and schedule.

Certain people might be more drawn to mosquitoes when they smelly armspits, according to studies. Researchers believe this could be one reason that some individuals appear to be particularly affected by reptiles, while other appear to be able to live completely unharmed.

The fatal malaria parasite is transported by mosquitoes and humans throughout the ages, and the first reports of this disease go back as far as 2700 B.C. The disease continues to affect humans and causes many thousands of people dying every year.

Over 110 countries have reported cases of malaria in the past, and Africa is the most affected with the highest death percentage (roughly 89 percent of deaths). Nearly half the population of the world lives in malaria-prone regions. Furthermore, children younger than five, pregnant women and those suffering from HIV/Helps are the most at risk for severe illness and death.

The story of malaria has seen many historical efforts to get rid of it. Quinine, an ingredient derived through the barks of cinchona tree, is identified as being effective against infected by the jungle from the 16th century onwards. When studying the way mosquitoes transmit malaria, scientists focused their attention on the control of vectors. They believed that by killing the vector, they would eliminate the disease's spread. This is why DDT as well as other insecticides were made widespread in the 19th century, and were used for decades afterward. A different method for controlling vectors which is not just effective however also cost-effective is using mattress nets that protect people asleep from being bit by mosquitoes.

Why does malaria remain an issue despite all the advancements in treatment? The main reason for worry is the rising incidence resistance to insecticides and medications. Natural selection favors certain varieties of malaria with genetic mutations that allow to ward off threats since they have been able to survive for over 50,000 years. Pests that resist medications and mosquitoes immune against insecticides have become more prevalent. International efforts are underway to combat fight against the disease of jungle fever: the development of malaria-specific vaccines which have the potential to save thousands of lives, and ultimately help in eradicating the effects of this abysmal disease.

The creation of an effective malaria vaccine poses an obstacle because of the complex life-cycle of Plasmodium. It is necessary to combine components targeting different life stages or the scientists must decide which stage of life the parasite is to focus on. But, new research has given the evidence that malaria vaccines could prove effective.

Malaria is distinct in comparison to many of illnesses we are as currently vaccine against due to that it does not exhibit sterile resistance. In the event that you are ill with the malaria and recover then you could be infected over and over. The immune system's response to malaria previously does not stop your from acquiring it once in the future. It's not like a condition such as measles. The majority of those who contract measles are not likely to contract the illness ever again. When it comes to malaria, there's evidence of a natural immunity. A person who was previously infected by the disease may develop it, but it's likely to be lesser severe. Because of this acquired immunity, the majority of people who contract malaria again in a number of African countries in which malaria is common experience slight signs. It is also the reason why intestinal illness is deadly for children under the age of five. Because of their inability to fight this parasite, children tend to experience a severe illness which could lead to deadly complications. Additionally, those who've never been exposed to malaria must be cautious as they might develop a fatal illness when they first get sick. In the end, a person who has developed insusceptibility isn't indefinitely. Actually the case of a person who lives in Africa and then leaves even one year, he is likely to lose the partially-protected status and will be just as vulnerable to malaria would someone who has never affected. So, the best way to approach establishing an effective malaria vaccine is to understand the concept of fractional resistance. This will allow the immunisation process in accordance with this conventional.

Clinical Trial Results for the Vaccine The latest clinical trials of the vaccine have yielded positive findings. The vaccine RTS,S has demonstrated as high as 50 percent efficacy for preventing malaria from youngsters. Even though this effectiveness rate may not be as impressive as we'd like it to be but it's an important step forward to fight against fever. As part of an extensive trial it is being tested in a variety of African countries.

Researchers have created an idea that was revealed during the review of 2002 that could lead to a variety of potential vaccines against the disease of the jungle. Most scientists employ technology to identify and then deliver certain antigens into vaccines instead of attempting to develop the live-attenuated vaccination. In addition, there are three distinct strategies for vaccines that are being researched in light of the parasite's 3 distinct life phases.

Pre-erythrocytic vaccinations focus on the infectious stage and seek to eliminate liver cells that are infected or stop sporozoites from entering the cells. The duration of the pre-erythrocytic vaccination is perhaps the greatest obstacle in less than one hour after the injection by mosquitoes, sporozoites enter the liver. This means that the parasite is removed swiftly through the body's immune system. Although the majority of potential pre-erythrocytic antibody are stage I or II, a vaccine is being tested in the Stage III stage of preliminaries, and provides a guarantee: RTS as well as the S vaccine. It's important to be aware that Stage III tests test efficacy and Phase I tests examine the safety.)

In the irradiated sporozoite study conducted in 2002 The RTS,S vaccine's creators determined the protein that is most responsible to protect. The circumsporozoite protein, also known as CS protein is the title for the antigen. While this protein is protective but it's not a particularly immunogenic in its own right, implying it's not great at triggering an immune response that is resistant. In the end, scientists used an antigen from the CS protein and the Hepatitis B surface antigen, which is the antigen responsible for protecting against infection in the Hepatitis B vaccine. A adjuvant, which is a chemical which boosts the immune system's reaction to the antigen, was employed by scientists to stimulate our immune system. To stop the pathogens causing the sporozoites to enter the liver cells and to determine particular infected cells to be destroyed High levels of antibodies have to be created.

Through Phase III studies, the vaccine RTS,S was evaluated across eleven African countries. Certain of the studies have proven positive. Initial findings that were released in October of 2011, demonstrated that infants aged between 5 and 17 months who had been vaccine-ed with RTSS, had 56 percent and 47% reduced likelihood of contracting clinical malaria or severe malaria, according to. The vaccine, however, proved less effective in the initial vaccination of infants who were who were between six and twelve weeks in accordance with the results of

November 2012. In the RTS,S vaccination group, there were the reduction of one third of cases of clinical and severe malaria for that class. The end-to-end results of the study, which surveyed the youngest children for a period of three years, revealed an increase of 26% for children who were the smallest and 36% for the children with clinical malaria up to 17 months of age at the time they had their first vaccine. In the European Medicines Agency recommended in July 2015 that this vaccine be authorized to be used within Africa in children as young as. The recommendation for vaccination is currently being considered by the World Health Organization. In the meantime, a WHO meeting on warnings has recommended testing the vaccine within 3-5 African countries of sub-Saharan. This is because the Malaria Vaccine Initiative, a non-profit organization with its headquarters within Seattle, Washington, is responsible for the development of RTS. In 2025, the organization is hoping to come up with a superior vaccine that will be more than 80 percent effective.

Researchers are working to boost the efficacy of the RTS,S vaccine up to over 50% with the help of the prime boost technology adjuvants, adjuvants, as well as optimizing the antigen. A variety of other vaccines for pre-erythrocytic disorders are under development and have not yet shown that same degree of success or effectiveness.

Erythrocytic vaccination or blood-stage vaccination will stop the rapid attack and the abiogenetic growth of the parasites in red platelets. Remember that this stage of blood is the first time symptoms begin to manifest and it is one of the most hazardous for patients as the red blood cells are expanding. The blood stage vaccine will be designed to limit the number of merozoites that infect red blood cells instead of entirely stop their reproduction because of the high quantity of merozoites created at this point (40,000 merozoites are released per every infected liver cell). Most blood-stage vaccinations remain being tested in Phase 1 or Phase II clinical trials. However, none have reached similar levels of effectiveness that the RTS and S vaccine has.

Not to be left out, an alternative type of vaccine targets the stomach phase in sexual reproduction. It aims to stop the spread of the parasite through killing the vector Anopheles mosquitoes the strategy is often known as the transmission-blocking vaccination (TBV). It's a nebulous method to combat the vaccination because it isn't able to ensure that a person is protected from the parasite, but will instead hinder the spreading process.

The vaccine Pfs25-EPA currently being developed through the Johns Hopkins University Center for Vaccine Research as well as the United States National Institute for Allergy & Infectious Diseases Lab of Malaria Immunology and Virology it is an TB vaccine potential candidate. The concept of the vaccination is that mosquitoes who consumes blood may take the antibodies in its stomach, if it has the ability to create antibodies against

Pfs25 antigen. In the stomach, these antibodies meet with the antigen, which allows them to block the parasite's growth and eliminate the parasite.

In the quest to create a malaria vaccine, many researchers believe the combination of different approaches could be the next stage. Whatever the case, single stage vaccines must prove their effectiveness on their own prior to allowing researchers to create that an immunisation join draws closer. In addition, the most important test that researchers are going to look into the upcoming tests is the fact that there aren't established resistance mechanisms or aversion, and there's nothing other than costly preliminary clinical tests on people to prove the effectiveness of an immunisation. So, even though substantial advances have been made making a malaria vaccine remain an expensive and complex undertaking.

How Malaria Vaccine Functions

Mosquirix is an "subunit" vaccine. It's because it has a tiny amount of a manufactured malaria parasite. The protein is paired by another "adjuvant", a particle designed to boost areas of force to initiate reactions. The main function of the vaccine is activating the body's ability to create antibodies that fight against parasites which kills it and hindering its entry into the liver cells. Once the parasite is in your body, it immediately attack those cells. In the event that a different area in the body's immune system responds to the vaccination, it also assists in triggering an inflammation reaction.

Controlling mosquito vectors, which is essentially stopping them from biting humans, or by killing mosquitoes or by using bed nets that are which are treated with insecticides--as well as diagnostics and treatment using medications to fight malaria are two strategies available to combat malaria as well as vaccination. Resistance to drugs, however, is an issue.

The world's most powerful malaria vaccine Mosquirix (generally known as RTS,S) was approved to use in the fight to fight Plasmodium falciparum malaria across Africa.

The vaccination works by preventing malaria parasites from getting into the liver, where it could grow and reproduce in order to trigger illness-related side effects.

The long-term effect of this vaccine hasn't been determined yet however, children ranging from five to 18 months had the greatest protection when the vaccine was given with three doses every month, and then followed by booster doses twenty months after.

Chapter 3: Measures To Avoid Mosquitoes

If you can avoid as many bites as is possible and avoiding them, you will greatly decrease the chance of contracting illnesses caused through insects. Moths don't just transmit malaria to people in tropical areas and dengue fever, but they also transmit malaria, Japanese encephalitis, and yellow fever. It is also possible to spread the disease by sandflies and ticks throughout the tropical region as well as elsewhere around the world. Most mosquitoes feed mostly at the dawn and night. Anopheles mosquitoes that carry malaria, feed during the night and can be active from sunset to dawn; Aedes mosquitoes, which transmit dengue fever and chikungunya are most active throughout the day (though they can bite during the night, especially in well-lit environments).

Some preventative measures include:

Wearing clothes and pants that have long sleeves at the times of risk (lighter colors are preferred over dark ones).

Beware of fragrances and perfumes as they can attract mosquitoes.

Use mosquito repellents that contain 30% DEET, Citriodiol (oil made from lemon eucalyptus (also known as PMD) or Picaridin on exposed skin, especially when you sweat or swim. Be sure to apply treatment on all exposed skin.

Do not sleep with the mosquito net is acceptable in the event that your lodging isn't covered or air-conditioned.

Infusing bedding, clothing, and bed nets with insecticide Permethrin

Vector Control

The phrase "vector control of malaria" is a term used to describe any method employed in order to eradicate or limit the spread of Anopheles mosquitoes, which carry malaria.

The most effective strategies to control malaria is through vector control. The Anopheles mosquito is the vector that transmits malaria. It is believed that they transmit the illness from animals to humans.

An insecticide to kill insects is applied every year, either once or twice across all surfaces in the home that mosquitoes may be a part of the indoor residual spray (IRS). The mosquitoes who enter homes have been found to be less likely to be able to survive because of this. The study estimates that 5percent of the in danger populations are protected by this method for controlling vectors.

Dependable insecticidal mosquito nets (LLIN) are nets for mosquitoes which are also sprayed with the insecticide. When it is nighttime, and the mosquito will be most likely bite, the nets serve as a physical and chemical shield for the mosquito. When utilized by large groups, they eliminate mosquitoes on a massive size.

Larviciding is the method using chemicals to destroy the larvae of mosquitoes to its breeding ground. The process works but only on areas where the mosquito breeding areas are centralized and readily accessible.

Major Obstacles to Malaria Control

Drug Resistance

At present, three of five malaria parasites that are human-affected have developed resistance to drugs. They include Plasmodium falciparum Plasmodium vivax, and Plasmodium malariae. If the malaria parasite is inaccessible to an antimalarial medication it takes the drug longer to kill each one of the parasites that reside in the body. This will take longer for a patient to stop experiencing the negative effects caused by diarrhea. The treatment may not remove all parasites from your body, in certain instances. The process of cross-resistance makes it more difficult to determine drug resistance. If a parasite is intolerant to a particular medication, it could become resistant to a second drug which functions similarly.

Cross Resistance

Many antimalarials have been taken entirely off the market due to they are no longer effective. One of the biggest threats for public health is the rise of Plasmodium falciparum, which is intolerant to the drug of choice artemisinin. Recent success in the global fight against malaria are mostly due to the combination of artemisinin treatment (ACTs). But the resistance to these therapies has emerged within Southeast Asia and is currently growing throughout this region of the globe.

The World Health Organization (WHO) issued a global plan in January of 2011 to tackle the rapidly growing problem of antimalarial resistance

Move the resistance in the areas that already have it or limit it.

Prevent the development of resistance to artemisininin within regions where it isn't currently a concern.

The public health implications could be devastating if the artemisinin-resistant is spread across Africa in the same way it has in the past with antimalarial medicines such as chloroquine. It is probable that the current reductions in the mortality rate of malaria could end up reversing.

To determine what genetic mutations within Plasmodium that are responsible for the resistance to artemisinin, scientists use whole genome sequencing, as well as different methods. Scientists may be able identify and possibly slow the progression of resistance in the event they identify the genetic mutations.

Insecticide Resistance

The capacity of insects to live and reproduce against an insecticide designed for killing it is commonly referred to as resistance against insecticides.

The control of malaria vectors is a challenge due to the fact that Anopheles mosquitoes have a resistance to insecticides. Resistance to insecticides occurs when some genetic change in the DNA of a mosquito allows it to survive encounter with an insecticide. This is similar to how malaria parasites are resistant to drugs that fight malaria. If the mosquitoes that remain develop, the genetic modification could be transmitted to the next generation and result in stronger mosquitoes. Anopheles mosquitoes were found to be intolerant to insecticides in 64 nations. Resistance to insecticides could cause an increased incidence of mortality and malaria cases in the event that it is not addressed. To prevent mosquitoes from becoming resistant different insecticides, methods are being devised to ensure they can be rotated on a regular basis. It is also hoped that innovative tools can be created to reduce the amount of mosquito vectors. In the case of mosquito populations, scientists are conducting whole genome sequences to pinpoint precisely which genes play a role in the resistance of insecticides.

Chapter 4: The Malaria Vaccine For Travel

The likelihood of contracting malaria among travelers will vary from one place from place to location, the time of the year, duration of stay, kind of accommodations, intensity of outdoor activity as well as other variables. Malaria usually isn't an investment at altitudes greater than 2,200 metres, however it can vary by country. Certain populations are more at risk of severe malaria Prior to making plans for travel to areas that are malaria-prone pregnant women, children and those who are younger than 5 are advised to be mindful of their risks.

It's more than bring you to a new place. It is a chance to get your energy back, widen the scope of your view, offer you an opportunity to explore something new, boost your imagination, and ultimately increase your happiness. The process of planning an excursion can be thrilling. There is a great deal of happiness and joy planning your trip and list your must-see places.

Booking appointments with a traveling doctor is one of the top things you can make prior to embarking on the road. Prior to and following their travels they assist in ensuring that travelers are happy as well as their safety. A visit to a specialist in traveling medicine is beneficial when planning your trip to another country. If, however, you're traveling to developing or underdeveloped nations that have more likelihood of contracting deadly transmissible diseases during your travels making an appointment at the travel clinic is crucial. People suffering from certain health conditions that reduce their immune systems, making them more prone to infection ailments also require it.

Every traveler should be vaccinated against influenza and are current on Coronavirus antibodies and their sponsors.

Additionally, it's important to adhere to the adult vaccination program, that includes:

Varicella, chickenpox and diphtheria and tetanus as well as pertussis (DTP) and pneumococcal. Mumps, measles as well as rubella (MMR) Polio and shingles.

What can we do to reduce your Risk of Malaria While traveling

Intestinal illness is a condition caused through an organism known as a parasite. The infection is spread through bites from mosquitoes that are contaminated. Antimalarial medicines can be used prior to traveling and during the duration of a stay as well as after return home after a certain duration. Travel medicine specialists is able to evaluate the advantages and disadvantages of each method of treatment or prevention. The medications to prevent malaria are offered. Chemoprophylaxis is the name for this. Chemoprophylaxis can eliminate malaria's blood stage and thus prevents symptoms of the disease. It is essential to use the antimalarial medication whenever you travel in an area that the possibility of getting malaria. They are able to lower the risk of contracting malaria nearly 90 percent.

Tips to stay healthy while travelling

Infection is among the most unpleasant things you can experience during a traveler. Verify the vaccinations as well as boosters are in good condition Also, get any new vaccinations recommended for the destination you are planning to visit.

If you are traveling, be sure to drink plenty of water and eat in a safe manner. Make sure to eat only cooked meals. Do not eat raw foods such as salads or raw veggies from streetside vendors. The only beverages that are bottled, and not just water, are recommended for consumption. This is particularly important when you plan to travel in areas that have little resources, such as Africa and Southeast Asia.

Chapter 5: Effect Of The Malaria Vaccine On The Global World

Over the last few years, numerous efforts have been undertaken in order to create compelling and rational anti-inflammation antibodies that can prevent intestinal illness. In the past ten years, there are a major milestone in the world's general health history because there's a global organization and responsibility of the world's benefactors, the public and private sector as well as research institutes, pharmaceutical firms and malariologist to tackle this deeply rooted hatred of human need by revitalizing the vital intestinal sickness vaccination inventive work that is focusing on the various types of intestinal illness parasites. In the end, several clinical trials are in progress across the globe, and preliminary results are positive and optimistic. In the present, scrutiny is more important and pertinent when you consider the current situation. This an effort to identify the challenges which are in place and to determine how experts in world public health are able to analyze and resolve the main problems and challenges which are in the present in order to lessen the burden of malaria around the world and, ultimately, eliminate it by providing vaccines that are safe and reliable. They are also efficient and inexpensive.

To reduce malaria's spread throughout communities and safeguard those who are given the vaccination Malaria vaccines are currently being created. The advancement in the immunization of intestinal illness is anticipated to yield a fruitful treatment of the disease known as jungle fever. Certain malarial immunisation newcomers have recently been identified and the genetic control of these predators has been proven to be more effective thanks to the advancement of modern biotechnology.

Ethical Considerations of the Malaria Vaccine

Research and management of malaria has been largely omitted the ethical aspects until recent. Even though this report offers a brief overview of the major problems to be addressed, more research is needed in a number of the mentioned subjects, in particular considering the fact that the field of malaria research, the epidemiology of malaria, as well as policy will likely alter in the near future.

The vast inequality with regard to risk for disease and outcomes for health is clearly evident by the rise of malaria. The awareness of this is a key component of recent advancements on control measures and financing initiatives. The people who are most in need of malaria controls are usually the ones who have the most difficulty accessing the same, as there are a lot of research gaps in the field of malaria as well as other related ailments. As with antimalarial resistance prevention, screening for mass populations programs and treatments, as well as the use of primaquine could be guided by ethical principles as well, treatments and the policy. When it comes to malaria research, explicit ethical guidelines should be formulated to ensure large-scale exploration efforts continue without imposing unnecessary risks on members. The ethical considerations will aid the successful and appropriate application of new techniques such as malaria vaccines and vectors that have been genetically altered with a view to the future. An encouraging development is the recent effort to increase capacity that have benefited local ethical expertise within endemic areas.

These preliminary studies are designed to spur further studies on ethical concerns related to malaria offer guidance for control protocols for evaluating the ethics of interventions as well as assist medical professionals, researchers as well as policymakers to pursue the goal of malaria-related control strategies which are ethically solid. Residents and patients of regions with high levels of malaria, most in require of ethically-designed programmes to combat malaria now and over the future are the final benefit of these efforts.

Challenges of Malaria Vaccine to Nations Development

As compared to the creation of different product types, such as small molecules, development of vaccines presents particular set of difficulties. As such, the process of assembling immunizations is innately a process of development and modification of living creatures, or parts of them, or the articulation of recombinant proteins in live cells. In spite of the fact that biological species are highly diverse, the process has to be optimized to ensure that vaccines are produced in a high-quality and efficient manner that can be commercially profitable. The altered protein or organism is required to be placed in a solution which is suitable for both oral or parenteral administration, and stabilizes the organism to provide the shelf-life of the product. Not least the analytical tests for defining the vaccination and ascertaining what is the "potency," or dose quantity, of the immunelogically active component(s) should be designed and tested.

These tasks could be a long time to accomplish due to their complexity and require coordination by experts in a wide range of disciplines.

Tragically, on the basis that the strains found in a random area are genetically and antigenically different and could occur during the course of an infection the patient should develop immunity to a handful of unique varieties and strains for complete protection. Due to repeated exposure the body can build up immunity rapidly in regions in which malaria is endemic in a matter of years while it can take longer for areas in which it's not as prevalent. The malaria vaccine that has the best profile remains several years from being achieved due to the intricate life-cycle, the specific immunologic and epidemiologic characteristics and the difficulties inherent to the development of vaccines. The possibility of eradicating malaria at a certain point in its life as well as the health goals of global scale to develop vaccines are the main drivers for the malaria vaccine's global approach to development. In the Malaria Vaccine Technology Roadmap calls to achieve the two following targets by the year 2030:

(1) The licensing of vaccinations against Plasmodium falciparum as well as Plasmodium Viralx, which have approximately 75% success against the disease in clinical settings and which are able to be carried out in a real-world setting as well (2) the development of vaccines which can be administered as large-scale campaign to prevent the spread of the parasite.

The development of vaccines is aimed that target different stages in the lifecycle of a parasite that include the pre-erythrocytic blood and sexual phases, all within the framework of the above goals. The most commonly targeted stage is the pre-erythrocytic period. A successful immunological and clinical method appears to stop the progression of erythrocytes and hepatocytes. Yet, there are other strategies that are being considered in parallel due to the limited RTS, S/AS01's efficiency. Its Controlled Human Infection Model (CHIM) is a model that permits new vaccines to be assessed to determine their efficacy as well as the immunologic correlates of protection through small-scale trials and then de-risked prior beginning large field studies This is a major advantage the malaria vaccine development group is able to offer over other vaccine development groups. Healthy people in this model are vaccinated which is then infected with malaria parasites, either through being bit by a mosquito or through injecting the sporozoites. Antimalarial medicines are utilized to treat infection and check the progress of malaria parasitemia within those who participate. The comparison of the rate of malaria among vaccine recipients as well as people who received placebo may give an indication early of the vaccine's efficiency.

Chapter 6: Causes Of Malaria

Malaria is a deadly and life-threatening illness that impacts millions around the world. The cause of the disease is an organism known as Plasmodium that is passed to humans by the bites of female Anopheles mosquitoes. In this section we'll have a more detailed review of the causes behind malaria as well as what is possible to do in order to help protect yourself from the deadly illness.

Environmental factors

The main cause of malaria is environmental. The mosquitoes that carry malaria flourish in hot and humid climates, and they are more frequent in regions with stagnant waters. They put their eggs into water. The larvae then develop within standing water, which makes the perfect breeding grounds for mosquitoes.

Human behaviour

Human behaviour also plays a part in transmitting malaria. Individuals who reside or work in locations with the highest risk of getting malaria are more likely develop the illness. It is the case for those who work in fields, or any some other outdoor spaces in which they are exposed to mosquitoes as well individuals who do not utilize mosquito nets or protection clothing to avoid the bites of mosquitoes.

Poor sanitation

Inadequate sanitation is yet another cause which contributes to the transmission of malaria. In the event that people do not have access to safe water or adequate sanitation facilities it is possible that they are more susceptible to contracting the illness. The reason for this is that mosquitoes reproduce in water that is dirty as well as the unsanitary environment can aid in parasites to transmit.

Insufficient immunity

In addition, a lack of immune system can also be a reason that could contribute to the growth of malaria. The people who reside in regions in which malaria is prevalent might develop an immunity to malaria in time. But, those who travel into these regions from non-endemic areas are more susceptible the illness because they've already accumulated immunity.

In general, malaria is due to a mixture of factors that affect the environment, our behavior, inadequate hygiene, and insufficient immunity. To prevent malaria, it's important to be aware of the dangers of bites from mosquitoes. For instance, applying mosquito nets and proper clothing and using insect repellent. Also, get medical help immediately when you notice signs of malaria such as headaches, fever, or muscle pains. With these measures and avoiding the risk of contracting malaria, you will reduce your chances of getting this devastating illness.

Parasites That Cause Malaria

The disease of malaria is brought on by a family of parasites called Plasmodium. The parasites transmit to human beings by the bites of female Anopheles mosquitoes. Here are the diverse kinds of parasites responsible for malaria and their effects on the human body.

Plasmodium falciparum

Plasmodium falciparum is among the most prevalent and fatal one of four types of Plasmodium which can are responsible for the spread of malaria to human beings. This is the cause of most deaths related to malaria all over the world.

If this parasite is introduced into in the bloodstream it swiftly expands and targets the blood red cells which causes them to split and let more parasites enter the bloodstream. The result is serious anemia and organ damage, which could be fatal if untreated.

Plasmodium vivax

Plasmodium Viax is the 2nd most prevalent kind of Plasmodium which causes malaria in human. In contrast to P. falciparum P. Vizax is able to remain dormant in the liver for a period of months or many years before being activated and causing another outbreak of malaria. The disease can become harder to control and treat.

Plasmodium malariae

Plasmodium malariae is an less widespread type of Plasmodium that can cause malaria in people. In contrast to P. falciparum or P. vixax, P. malariae does do not cause serious disease or even death, however it could cause persistent infections that may be long-lasting if untreated.

Plasmodium ovale

Plasmodium ovale is one of the less widespread kind of Plasmodium which causes malaria in humans. It's similar to P. virax in the sense that it has the ability to lie in the liver and dormant for prolonged periods before it reactivates and causes symptoms.

The malaria parasites are a family of four types of Plasmodium that can be transmitted to people through bites of mosquitoes infected. The parasites cause various symptoms that range that range from mild to extreme that can result in serious illness or even death in the event of not being treated. To safeguard yourself against malaria, you need to be aware of the dangers of mosquito bites. This includes making use of insect nets or a protective clothes, and applying repellents for insects. Also, get medical help immediately when you notice signs of malaria, like headaches, fever, or muscle pains. With these measures and avoiding the risk of contracting malaria, you will reduce your chances of getting this devastating illness.

Transmission Of Malaria

In the event that an infected female mosquito bites someone she injects Plasmodium parasites into the bloodstream. The parasites travel on to the liver, and there they start to multiply and grow. In a short time they leave the liver, and then enter the bloodstream where they affect the red blood cells.

The parasites grow in those red blood cells the cells explode and release more parasites into bloodstream. This can trigger a variety of signs, such as headache, fever as well as muscle pain.

Preventing Malaria Transmission

One of the best ways to avoid the spread of malaria is to stay away from being bit by mosquitoes infected. You can do this through the use of mosquito nets, wearing long sleeves, and applying repellents to your skin. Also, it is important to get rid of any water sources that are stagnant around the workplace or at home since they can serve as the breeding ground for mosquitoes.

If you're traveling to an area where there is the highest risk of suffering from malaria, you must make additional preparations. For instance, you could take medications to prevent malaria, staying in mosquito nets and wearing clothing that is protective. It is also recommended to get medical help promptly if you notice any signs of malaria. the early detection and treatment could aid in stopping the illness from becoming more widespread.

Alongside these steps in tackling the mosquito population with spraying insecticide and other strategies could also reduce transmission of malaria within the affected regions.

Chapter 7: Symptoms Of Malaria

Although some patients with malaria might not show any signs while others might experience various symptoms which can be minor to serious. The following are common signs of malaria as well as what to do if suspect you might suffer from malaria.

Fever

The most frequent signs associated with malaria is fever that ranges from mild to extremely. It usually is experienced in a series of that cause chills. This is followed by rapid increase in temperature and sweating. The fever can be experienced on a daily basis for diseases due to Plasmodium virax and Plasmodium ovale or three days for those suffering from infections brought on through Plasmodium malariae. In certain cases there is a possibility that the fever could remain constant and not have the pattern of cyclic.

Headache and Body Aches

A common sign of malaria is headache, and it is often severe and debilitating. Joint pains and joint pains are also common, and often coupled with fatigue and weak. This can cause difficult to complete everyday activities, and can be present for many days.

Nausea and Vomiting

Vomiting and nausea are typical symptoms of malaria especially in young children. The symptoms can occur as an outcome of flu and could result in dehydration if it is not addressed quickly.

Other Symptoms

Alongside these typical signs, those suffering from malaria can also suffer from different symptoms such as nausea, cough and breathing difficulties. If the malaria is severe, it may cause complications like anemia, organ failure and the death.

If you believe you be suffering from malaria, it's essential to get medical attention immediately. An early diagnosis and treatment will aid in stopping the illness from advancing and lower the likelihood of complications. Treatment usually involves a regimen of antimalarial medications, which may differ based upon the kind of parasite that causes the disease and the intensity of signs.

Complications Of Malaria

Although many individuals can recover from malaria after proper treatment, malaria can result in serious complications. Here are some issues with malaria that you must be conscious of.

Cerebral Malaria

Cerebral malaria is a very rare yet severe form of malaria which is affecting the brain. It's more prevalent for pregnant and young children. Signs of cerebral malaria can include seizures, confusion and complications such as coma. This condition can lead to death when not addressed promptly.

Anemia

Anemia is one of the most common complications of malaria. It is most prevalent among pregnant women and infants. Anemia is a condition that occurs when the body doesn't have enough red blood cells deliver oxygen to the tissues. This could cause an increase in fatigue, weakness and shortness of breath.

Kidney Failure

Sometimes it can result in kidney insufficiency. It occurs when kidneys are not able to clear the excess fluid and waste from the body. The signs of kidney failure could include swelling, blood pressure, or decreased urinary output.

Respiratory Distress

Malaria is also a cause of breathing problems, especially among children. The complication could cause trouble breath, rapid respiration and chest discomfort. If it is severe breathing problems can cause life-threatening complications.

Low Blood Sugar

Malaria is known to cause a decline of blood sugar levels especially in youngsters. A drop in blood sugar could cause fatigue, dizziness and confusion.

Pregnancy Complications

The malaria virus can cause problems during pregnancy, which include preterm birth and low birth weight as well as stillbirth. The pregnant women are especially susceptible to malaria and need steps to avoid infections.

For conclusion, though some people do recuperate from malaria using appropriate treatments, malaria can lead to serious complications. They can pose a life-threatening threat and need immediate medical treatment. If you've just traveled to an area that is at risk or you are suffering from signs of malaria, you should get medical attention immediately in order to stop the illness from advancing and creating complications. Preventing malaria is essential, therefore make sure you are protected from bites by mosquitoes. Also, follow suggested prevention guidelines if have traveled to a highly-risk zone.

Long-Term Effects Of Malaria

Although most people are able to are able to recover from malaria after proper treatment, malaria can be long-lasting and affect people. Here are a few chronic effects of malaria are worth knowing about.

Neurological Effects

The malaria virus can cause a wide range of neurological symptoms in certain individuals, especially those who have experienced frequent or severe instances of the illness. The effects could include seizures, confusion and problems with speech or movement. In very rare instances malaria, it can cause permanent brain injury.

Anemia

Anemia is the most common complication of malaria. It is most prevalent among pregnant women and infants. If untreated anemia may lead to permanent health complications such as weakening, fatigue as well as cognitive impairment.

Organ Damage

The effects of malaria can affect many organs within the body, like the kidneys, liver, and the spleen. If not treated it can lead to permanent harm to organs that are damaged, which can lead to chronic health issues like kidney or liver insufficiency.

Recurrent Infections

The disease can lead to chronic infections, most notably for those who reside in areas where malaria is the most prevalent. The recurrence of infections could cause chronic health issues including cognitive impairment, anemia as well as other health issues that last for a long time.

In the end, although many have the ability to overcome malaria after proper treatment, malaria can result in long-term consequences for some people. They can be a result of neurologic issues to damage to organs as well as recurring illnesses. If you've had previously experienced malaria or have symptoms associated with the condition, you need to seek medical treatment in order to stop long-term health issues from arising. Preventing is the best way to stay healthy, so make sure you are protected from bites by mosquitoes. Also, take the necessary precautions in the event that you're traveling to an area that has a high risk of malaria.

Chapter 8: Diagnosis Of Malaria

The early diagnosis and timely diagnosis are crucial to avoid serious complications as well as decreasing the chance of transmitting. In this section we'll look at the diverse methods employed to diagnose malaria.

Symptoms and Medical History

The first step for diagnosing malaria is to look at the patient's symptoms as well as the medical background. Most malaria cases are accompanied by headaches, fever, or flu-like symptoms. If you've been to or reside in the area that is prone to malaria the doctor you see will be very suspicious of this disease.

Blood Tests

The most popular method for diagnosing malaria is to perform a blood test. There are two kinds of tests for blood: microscopical examination as well as Rapid testing for diagnostics (RDTs).

Microscopic Examination

A microscopic exam requires taking a portion from the blood of the patient and then examining it with an microscope to determine the malaria parasite. This is considered to be as the best method to diagnose malaria because it's extremely precise and also identify the type of parasite.

Rapid Diagnostic Tests (RDTs)

Diagnostic tests that are rapid (RDTs) can be used as an alternative to microscopically-based examination. The tests use only a small amount of blood, and can deliver results within 15 to 20 minutes. They're not as accurate as microscopy, but they are widely accepted as reliable and are employed in regions with minimal lab resources.

Molecular Tests

Tests using molecular methods, like Polymerase Chain Reaction (PCR) are extremely sensitive and precise in identifying malaria parasites. They are able to detect extremely small amounts of parasite as well as differentiate between species. But, molecular tests can be more costly and require special laboratory equipment and skilled technicians.

Prevention and Treatment

Preventing is the best way to avoid malaria. There are a number of methods for avoiding mosquito bites. If you're planning to travel to an area that has a high risk of malaria you must wear precautions like long sleeves and a t-shirt as well as mosquito nets as well as applying repellent for insects.

If you've been diagnosed with malaria, timely intervention is essential to avoid grave complications. Treatment usually involves a mixture of antimalarial drugs, and the exact regimen is contingent on the extent of the illness as well as the kind of parasite.

The treatment of malaria depends upon a mix of symptoms as well as medical histories and lab tests. Tests for blood, which include microscopy and quick diagnostic tests are among the most frequently used tests to determine the severity of the illness. These tests are very specific and precise, however they cost more and need special lab equipment. Preventing the spread of malaria. Getting treatment promptly is essential to avoid serious problems. If you've traveled to an area with a high risk of malaria and have symptoms of malaria, it's essential to seek medical attention promptly.

Differential Diagnosis Of Malaria

Malaria-related symptoms may be similar to the symptoms associated with other illnesses, which makes it difficult to identify. Here are some of the possible treatment options for malaria, which includes other diseases with similar symptoms.

Dengue Fever

Dengue fever can be described as a virus which is transmitted through mosquitoes. Similar to malaria, the dengue virus could result in headaches, fever, joint and muscle pain as well as fatigue. In certain cases, dengue fever can also result in a mild rash or bleeding. Dengue fever is most common in cities and frequent in tropical regions that include Southeast Asia and Latin America.

Typhoid Fever

Typhoid fever is a illness caused by the bacteria Salmonella Typhi. The symptoms of typhoid flu are akin to malaria. These include headaches, fever and muscle pains. It can also lead to stomach pain, diarrhea as well as a skin rash. Typhoid fever occurs most commonly in regions with low sanitation and hygiene. Moreover, the disease is common in regions in Africa, Asia, and South America.

Influenza

Influenza, sometimes referred to as the flu is a respiratory illness brought on by the virus influenza. Influenza's symptoms are similar to the symptoms of malaria. They include headaches, fever, tension, and fatigue. It can also lead to sore throats, coughs and nasal congestion. Influenza is more prevalent in warmer climates, and it is widespread throughout the world.

Viral Hepatitis

Viral hepatitis refers to a variety of infections caused by viruses which can result in liver inflammation. The symptoms of viral liver disease are similar to those of malaria. These include fatigue, fever, and muscle pains. The virus can cause nausea, abdominal pain and vomiting. The incidence of viral hepatitis is higher in places with poor hygiene and sanitation, but it's prevalent throughout the world.

Chapter 9: Medications And Therapies For Treating Malaria

There are a variety of treatments and medications readily available to effectively fight malaria. In this section we'll discuss various treatments and medications employed to treat malaria.

Antimalarial Medications

Antimalarial drugs are the mainstay of treatment for malaria. The selection of the medication is based on the type of Plasmodium parasite responsible for the disease and the extent of the disease, as well as the medical history and age that the individual sufferer has.

Artemisinin-based Combination Therapy (ACT)

ACT is the treatment recommended for malaria that is not complicated and due to Plasmodium falciparum. It is an amalgamation of artemisinin and another medicine that's taken for three days. ACT is extremely efficient and has greatly contributed in reducing deaths due to malaria worldwide.

Chloroquine

Chloroquine can be a very effective treatment for malaria that is not complicated due to Plasmodium vix as well as Plasmodium ovale. Also, it is used to treat prevention of malaria in areas that have these species. However, chloroquine-resistant strains of Plasmodium falciparum are widespread, so it is no longer recommended for treating this species.

Quinine

Quinine is a more traditional medication which was the primarystay of treatment for malaria. Quinine is used to treat complex or severe malaria, and often in combination with antibiotics. Quinine is known to cause side negative effects such as tinnitus nausea and headache.

Other Medications

Other antimalarial medications used for treating malaria include atovaquone-proguanil, mefloquine, and doxycycline. These medicines are employed as a prophylaxis treatment or to treat certain types of malaria.

Therapies

As well as medication, there are a number of treatments employed to aid in the treatment for malaria.

Fluids and Electrolytes

The severe malaria condition can lead to electrolyte imbalances and dehydration. People suffering from severe malaria might require intravenous fluids or the replacement of electrolytes.

Blood Transfusions

Acute malaria may cause anemia and may necessitate blood transfusions. The transfusion of blood can also be necessary for those suffering from grave complications, for example serious jaundice or cerebral malaria.

It is crucial to see a doctor if there is a suspicion that you are suffering from malaria or another serious disease. A prompt diagnosis and timely treatment will increase your odds for a complete recuperation.

Combination Therapies For Malaria

Combination treatments for malaria relate to the usage of multiple medications for treating malaria-related infections. The treatment is recommended by the World Health Organization (WHO) as the most effective treatment option for mild malaria because they lower the chance of developing resistance to medication and boost the efficacy of the treatment.

Malaria is caused by Plasmodium parasite, which is carried through mosquitoes. The illness affects millions people across the globe, with a particular focus on Sub-Saharan Africa in which it is the leading reason for mortality and morbidity. Malaria symptoms include headaches, fever, muscle discomfort, fatigue and muscle along with other signs. If not treated the malaria condition can develop into serious illness, and may be life-threatening.

Antimalarial medicines are employed to treat malaria-related infections. They can be classified into various categories, such as artemisinins other quinolines and antifolates. The most common combination therapies comprise artemisinin-based medicines that are fast-acting and efficient against a broad variety of Plasmodium species. There is also the drug of a companion, which is longer-lasting and lowers the chance that recrudescence (reappearance of parasites within the blood following treatment).

Combination therapies based on artemisinin (ACTs) are suggested by the WHO as the primary treatment for mild malaria brought on via Plasmodium falciparum, a dangerous strain of Plasmodium. ACTs are proven to be extremely reliable and safe as cure rates exceed 95percent. Utilization of ACTs have also led to an increase in deaths from malaria all over the world.

Examples of ACTs include artemether lumefantrine, artesunate amodiaquine and artesunate-mefloquine. The drugs are generally administered by mouth once a day for 3 days. They are usually well tolerated. The adverse effects tend to be minor and may include headache nausea, dizziness and nausea.

Other combination therapies used for malaria treatment include sulfadoxine-pyrimethamine, which is used as intermittent preventive treatment in pregnant women and infants, and chloroquine-primaquine, which is used for the treatment of malaria caused by Plasmodium vivax and Plasmodium ovale.

Intravenous Therapies For Severe Malaria

Intravenous treatments for the treatment of severe malaria refers to the administration of antimalarial medications which are administered directly to the bloodstream via the vein. Severe malaria can be a fatal illness that may result in multi-organ dysfunction and even death if not treated. Intravenous treatments are an essential part of managing extreme malaria. They're typically given in a hospital environment under the supervision of a physician.

Severe malaria is typically due to Plasmodium falciparum, which is the most deadly kind of Plasmodium. The signs of severe malaria are excessive fever, disorientation seizures, seizures and organ failure, in addition to many others. Rapid diagnosis and timely treatment are crucial to avoid complications and deaths.

Intracavenous treatments for malaria that are severe usually involve the drugs based on artemisinin, which have high efficacy and are swiftly working. The drugs are artesunate quinine and artemether as well as other things. The intravenous treatment is preferable to oral treatment in extreme malaria patients due to the potential for poor absorption, decreased consciousness as well as vomiting.

Artesunate is the most commonly used drug for treating serious malaria, according to World Health Organization (WHO) guidelines. It's highly effective having a cure rate of as high as 90 percent as well as being proven to lower mortality in extreme malaria instances. Artesunate typically is used as a daily intravenous injection for 3 days. Then, it is administered as an oral treatment for a period of 7 days.

The two drugs are alternate treatment options for serious malaria however, they can cause higher risk of adverse side effects than artesunate. Artemether typically is used as a daily intravenous infusion over three days. Then, it is and then oral therapy is followed for seven days. Quinine is given via intravenous infusions every eight hours over 7 consecutive days which is and then followed by oral therapy for seven consecutive days.

Treatments for malaria that are intravenous may cause adverse consequences, such as hypotension, irregular electrolyte levels, and cardiac arrhythmias among others. Monitoring of patients closely is crucial to control these issues.

For the record the fact that intravenous therapy is essential to managing severe malaria. It is a deadly illness that may result in multi-organ dysfunction and ultimately death if it is not addressed. Artesunate is the most commonly used drug to treat extreme malaria. It can be extremely efficient in decreasing mortality rates. Quinine and artemether are both other alternatives, but both can have more detrimental side effects. Monitoring of patients closely is vital to prevent risks of complications from intravenous therapy.

Chapter 10: Natural And Home Remedies For Managing Malaria Symptoms

Medical treatment is vital to manage the symptoms of malaria, there's certain home remedies that could assist in relieving signs and strengthen the immune system of your body.

Herbal Tea

Herbal teas like ginger, chamomile and peppermint are able to help lower headaches and fever that are caused by malaria. They have anti-inflammatory as well as analgesic qualities that help alleviate body pain and the discomfort.

Grapefruit

Drinking grapefruit juice or its pulp will help to reduce the signs of malaria. Grapefruit has compounds resembling quinine that could help reduce the malaria-related fever.

Turmeric

Turmeric is an effective antioxidant and anti-inflammatory spice that helps boost the immune system as well as reduce inflammation. The consumption of turmeric tea, or the addition of the spice to your meals may help alleviate effects of malaria, and also boost general well-being.

Coconut Water

Coconut water is a great natural source of electrolytes as well as nutrients which help your body to recover from the negative consequences of malaria. It is a great way to replenish liquids that are lost because of sweating and fever. It could assist in the reduction of nausea and vomiting that are associated to the illness.

Papaya Leaves

Papaya leaves are full of enzymes which could boost your immune system as well as reduce signs of malaria. The juice of the leaf or tea made from leaves may help lower the inflammation and fever caused by the illness.

It is vital to keep in mind that although home remedies may aid in relieving the symptoms of malaria they shouldn't be utilized to replace medical care. If you think you are suffering from malaria, it's essential to get medical treatment promptly. It can be a serious life-threatening illness, and immediate medical attention is essential to ensure a speedy recovery.

Herbal Medicines For Malaria

Herbal remedies have been utilized over the centuries to treat diverse range of diseases such as malaria. A lot of herbs possess antimalarial qualities and can assist in the prevention and treatment of illness. Below are some herbs which have been utilized to treat malaria-related symptoms:

Artemisinin

Artemisinin is a chemical that is derived of the Artemisia annua plant. It is also called sweet wormwood. It is among the most potent herbal remedies used to treat malaria.

Combination therapies based on artemisinin (ACTs) are extensively utilized to treat malaria that is not complicated and have been shown to be extremely effective.

Cinchona Bark

Cinchona bark has been identified as the main source for quinine, the first antimalarial medicine. It has been utilized throughout the ages for treating malaria, and continues to be used in some areas in the world for an herbal remedy. Cinchona bark has alkaloids in it that aid in reducing the chills and fever related to malaria.

Neem

Neem is a herb that is native to India which has been utilized over the years to treat a variety of ailments, such as malaria. Neem leaves are a source of compounds which can lower fever and ease inflammation.

Ginger

Ginger is a powerful natural anti-inflammatory that can reduce inflammation and discomfort that are associated with malaria. Also, it is antiviral and antibacterial properties that can boost the immune system while fighting from infections.

Garlic

Garlic contains antimalarial qualities and is utilized for many years in treating the illness. It is rich in compounds that aid in reducing chills, fever as well as other signs of malaria.

Even though herbal medicine may be beneficial in controlling the symptoms of malaria, it's vital to see a doctor when you suspect you may have malaria. It can be a serious or life-threatening condition, so timely medical attention is essential for the successful healing. Herbal remedies should be taken with care and with the advice of a health professional in order in order to stay clear of potential negative side negative effects as well as interactions with other medicines.

Nutritional Strategies For Managing Malaria

Antimalarial medicines are often the main treatment option of malaria, diet plays a vital aspect in managing the disease. Below are some strategies for nutrition to help control symptoms of malaria

Hydration Malaria can lead to dehydration, therefore it's important to drink a lot of fluids to keep yourself hydrated. Drinking water is the most effective option however coconut water, fruit juices and herbal teas are also hydrolyzing.

Vitamin C: Vitamin C is an antioxidant with potent properties which can lower inflammation and improve immunity. Vitamin C-rich foods are orange fruits and berries mangoes, kiwis and papayas.

Zinc: Zinc is an important mineral that helps strengthen the immune system as well as help reduce inflammation. The foods that contain zinc are fish, meat, nut seeds, whole grains.

Iron Malaria may cause anemia and it's important to keep your iron levels healthy. Iron-rich food items comprise of fish, meat and poultry, as well as lentils, beans, as well as refined cereals.

Anti-inflammatory food items: Malaria can cause inflammation within the body. Therefore, eating foods that are anti-inflammatory can alleviate symptoms. Diets that contain anti-inflammatory ingredients are fruits, vegetables and seeds, as well as nuts as well as fatty fish.

Probiotics: These are beneficial bacteria that are found in the stomach and are able to help boost our immune system. Foods that are rich in probiotics include yogurt, kefir sauerkraut and kimchi as well as Kombucha.

Nutrition can be helpful in managing the symptoms of malaria, it's important to get medical help in the event that you think you may have malaria. The disease can be severe and life-threatening illness, so timely medical attention is essential to ensure that you recover. The nutritional strategies must be utilized in conjunction with antimalarial medicines with the help by a medical professional in order to make sure that you are taking the best care of the illness.

Chapter 11: Preventing Malaria

(Tips for Staying Safe in High-Risk Areas)

If you plan to go to a highly-risk region, taking preventative steps are essential in order to prevent your body from getting the illness. Here are some guidelines to stay safe in highly-risk zones and for avoiding malaria:

Applying insect repellent can prevent mosquito bites. These are the main cause of transmission for malaria. Select a repellent with at the minimum of 20 percent DEET Apply it on your clothing and skin.

Dress in protective clothes: Covering the skin with long sleeves and trousers can prevent bites by mosquitoes. Light-colored clothes can aid in repelling mosquitoes as they are drawn to dark-colored clothing.

You can sleep beneath a mosquito net The mosquito net could create a physical barrier between your body and mosquitoes. It is important to ensure that the net is coated with insecticides and completely covers your mattress.

Utilize air conditioning. In the event of mosquito bites, they are less likely to get into rooms with air conditioning, and having fans or air conditioning will help to prevent bites from mosquitoes.

Use antimalarial medications: If you're traveling to an area that has a high risk of malaria in the United States, taking antimalarial medication prior to as well as after your travels can prevent malaria. It is important to speak with your physician about what the most effective antimalarial medication is for you.

Get rid of standing water. The mosquitoes reproduce in standing water So removing standing water surrounding your home will help to prevent the spread of mosquitoes.

Keep your indoors clear of the sun at dawn and dusk. The mosquitoes are at their most active during dawn and dusk. Therefore, being indoors at these times could reduce the possibility of getting mosquito bites.

Take care of yourself if you are experiencing symptoms such as symptoms like headache, chills, fever or body aches following having returned from an area of high risk Seek medical attention as soon as you can. It is a serious life-threatening illness, and urgent medical care is vital for the successful healing.

Protective Clothing And Gear For Malaria Prevention

Wearing protective clothing and equipment is vital to prevent malaria, specifically in highly-risk zones in which mosquitoes carrying malaria are widespread. The right clothes and accessories can decrease the chance of getting mosquito bites and help prevent malaria's spread. Here are some guidelines on how to select and wear protection gear and clothing to help prevent malaria

The pants and long-sleeved shirts Long-sleeved clothing such as clothing and pants may aid in protecting your skin from bites of mosquitoes. Select lightweight, breathable and comfortable fabrics like cotton as they're comfortable when you live in humid and hot climates.

Dark-colored clothes: Mosquitoes tend to be attracted by dark-colored colors and light colors, therefore wearing clothing that is lighter in color helps to decrease your visibility to the insects.

Clothing that repels insects: Insect clothing that is repellent is coated with permethrin, which is a chemical insecticide, which repels mosquitoes. The clothing works well in repelling mosquito bites and it can be cleaned and reused many times.

Nets for the head: These nets can be essential to protect your neck and face from bites by mosquitoes. They're especially useful while relaxing or sleeping outdoors.

Mosquito nets- Mosquito nets can be a great method to shield yourself from mosquito bites during your sleep. The nets should be treated by insecticide and covered with whole sleeping space.

The use of socks and shoes socks and shoes can to protect your feet from bites by mosquitoes. The mosquitoes love feet, which is why it's essential to wear shoes with closed toes as well as socks that are padded to protect the ankles of your feet.

Hands covered: If working in risky zones, gloves will aid in protecting your hands from insect bites.

Important to keep in mind the fact that protective gear and clothing must be utilized in conjunction in conjunction with preventive methods, such like insect repellents or antimalarial drugs. In addition, it is essential that you follow the directions of the manufacturer for insect repellents and clothing treated with insecticides.

Chapter 12: The Role Of Vaccines In Preventing And Treating Malaria

Despite the significant advancements in decreasing malaria's impact however, malaria is still a significant health problem, with the greatest impact in sub-Saharan African. The most efficient method to fight malaria is using insecticide-treated bed nets as well as spraying residuals in the indoor environment; scientists are researching vaccines that could offer long-term protection from the malaria.

Development of a successful malaria vaccine has proven to be a challenge because of the complexity of the malaria parasite as well as how it interacts with our immune system. In recent times there have been substantial improvements in the malaria vaccine research as well as several potential vaccines are in various stages of testing in clinical.

The most sophisticated malaria vaccine option is RTS/AS01 which was developed by GlaxoSmithKline together with the PATH Malaria Vaccine Initiative. RTS,S/AS01 is an recombinant protein vaccine which targets the circumsporozoite proteins (CSP) which is which is a protein that can be located on the outer surface of malaria parasites. It also includes an adjuvant called AS01 which increases the immune response towards the CSP antigen.

Research on RTS,S/AS01 has demonstrated that the vaccine offers only a small amount of protection against malaria among the infants of Africa. In a vast-scale Phase III trial conducted in various African nations it was discovered that the vaccine is able to lower the prevalence of chronic malaria by 39% for young children between 5 and 17 months old, and 27% for babies aged between 6 and 12 weeks. It was also discovered to lower the prevalence of malaria severe by 29% among young children between 5 and 17 months old, and 15% for babies aged between 6 and 12 weeks.

A potential malaria vaccine is the R21/MatrixM vaccine that was created by scientists from The University of Oxford and Novavax. R21/Matrix is a protein subunit vaccine targeting the CSP antigen. It's as is RTS,S/AS01. The difference is that the R21 vaccine contains a distinct adjuvant, called Matrix M, that has been demonstrated to increase immunity to CSP antigen.

Initial results from the Phase IIb clinical trial for R21/MatrixM carried out at Burkina Faso showed that the vaccine offered as much as 77% of immunity against malaria that is clinically prevalent among children aged 5 to 36 months. It also revealed that the vaccine was well tolerated and had a high security health profile.

Chapter 13: Combating Malaria

(Global Efforts and Future Directions)

Based on the World Health Organization (WHO) the WHO estimates there were 229 million malaria cases globally in the year 2019, and forty nine thousand deaths, mainly of children under the age of five in Africa sub-Saharan. In the last decade, substantial improvements have been made towards the reduction of the burden caused by malaria. The numbers show the reduction of 21% in the incidence of malaria as well as a decrease of 31% in the mortality rate for malaria between 2010 and the year 2019.

Global malaria elimination programmes include collaboration efforts between international agencies, governments and local communities to eliminate malaria throughout the world. The programs employ a wide range of tactics, which include the dispersal of insecticide-treated bednets as well as indoor residual spraying for the diagnosis and treatment of patients as well as studies and the creation of new methods.

The most efficient ways to combat malaria and elimination is through the use for insecticide-treated beds nets (ITNs). They can help stop mosquito bites as well as lower the likelihood of transmission. The WHO advises that everyone susceptible to malaria rest in ITNs and especially pregnant women as well as children. Between between 2010 and 2019, the number of people who are who are at risk of getting malaria in ITNs has increased from 30% to 46% worldwide and significant increase in Africa sub-saharan, where there is the greatest prevalence of malaria.

A different strategy to aid in eliminating malaria is the indoor residual spraying (IRS) that involves spraying insecticides onto the ceilings and walls of the houses to eliminate mosquitoes responsible for transmitting malaria. IRS is proven to cut down on malaria transmission up to 90%. However, the effectiveness of this method is dependent on quality of the insecticides used as well as trained staff as well as the participation of communities.

The early diagnosis and timely treatment for malaria-related cases is essential for the prevention of acute illness and decreasing transmission. Diagnostic tests that are rapid (RDTs) are commonly utilized in countries that are malaria-endemic for detecting any malaria-related parasites present in blood sample. Combination therapies based on artemisinin (ACTs) provide the most effective method of treating mild malaria. They have also contributed to a decrease of mortality from malaria in the past few years.

Despite impressive advancements in malaria elimination, programs have many hurdles to overcome, which include lack of funding, resistance to drugs as well as insecticide resistance. insufficient health infrastructures. Additionally, the spread of malaria can be influenced by environmental economic, and social aspects, which makes it challenging to manage in certain areas.

In order to overcome these obstacles to overcome these challenges, worldwide malaria elimination programs have to be sustained, well supported, and adapted to the local environment. Development and research into new techniques and treatments like the latest generation of insecticides, drugs as well as vaccines, are vital in achieving the goals of malaria elimination. A strong community participation model, healthy health systems and multisectoral cooperation are essential to achieve successful implementation.

Innovative Approaches To Malaria Prevention And Treatment

The spread of malaria remains an important public health problem all over the world, with a significant impact on deaths and morbidity, especially in the countries of low income. Despite numerous efforts to stop the spread of malaria innovative strategies are required to prevent and effectively treat this disease. There are many creative strategies currently being designed to fight malaria.

A promising method for malaria prevention involves the utilization of mosquitoes that have been genetically altered. Researchers are studying the use of modified mosquitoes with genetic modifications which are not susceptible to malaria or contain genes that render their chances less favourable to transmit virus to humans. The mosquitoes may be released into the wild in order to decrease the total amount of mosquitoes carrying malaria.

A different strategy to prevent malaria is to use novel insecticides. The traditional insecticides, like DDT were employed for a long time in order to prevent the spread of malaria however, the insect population is getting resistant to these chemical. Researchers are in the process of developing novel efficient insecticides that are not as harmful to human beings as well as the surrounding ecosystem.

As well as the use of new insecticides, scientists are investigating the possibility of using botanical extracts of plants in order to stop and combat malaria. In particular, artemisinin an ingredient found in the Artemisia annua plant is used as a component in treatments to treat malaria. Researchers are currently studying additional phytochemicals that may have antimalarial effects.

Innovative technologies, like mobile phone apps and remote sensing, are utilized to prevent and treat malaria. In particular, mobile apps for phones are able to monitor the spread the illness and warn health professionals of potential instances of outbreaks. Technologies for remote sensing could be employed to determine locations where malaria-carrying insects tend to breed, and allow an effective and targeted approach to controlling malaria.

Apart from the technological advancements in malaria prevention, there are other strategies that are economic and social in the prevention and management of malaria. Examples include initiatives that supply beds nets treated with insecticides for vulnerable groups have proved efficient in reducing the frequency of malaria. The campaigns for education and awareness can aid in stopping the spread of malaria.

In the end, there are a variety of creative strategies to combat malaria and treatment currently being researched and developed. Research and investment into these methods will be vital for the worldwide effort to end malaria as a health risk.

Chapter 14: The Life Cycle Of The Mosquito

While all mosquito species need standing water for reproduction however, they are found across a range of environments. Certain mosquito species are known to "floodwater" species because they reproduce in unstable aquatic environments and other mosquito species are known as "permanent water" species because they reproduce in permanent aquatic habitats. The evolution of other species is so specific that they only lay eggs in man-made or natural containers.

Every mosquito goes through the same life-cycle of four stages including egg, larva pupa, and matures The stages of pupa and larva behaving as if they were in the water, irrespective of the location they prefer to breed in.

Mosquito Eggs

The species that is responsible for the eggs will determine the female mosquito may deposit her eggs in one spot at a time, or in groups that are linked, known as rafts. Eggs are laid directly on the surface of still water or along the edges, within tree holes, or any other locations that are susceptible to floods from rainfall, water, or any other natural catastrophes. The temperature can affect the eggs' development and the species, eggs could hatch within a couple of days from the time they are laid. The exact timing will depend upon the specific species. In contrast in the event that the egg was laid without water and periodically submerged and flooded, it may stay inactive for several years prior to the natural conditions for hatching occur. Though some species of mosquitoes might overwinter as larvae, or adults, they typically stay during the egg stage.

The stage of the larva.

Larval stage begins as soon as the egg is born. Since they need air to breathe, larvae of most mosquito species hang suspended in the water's surface. From the rear of the larva up toward the water's surface an air tube, also known as a siphon acts as snorkel. The larvae that feed on filtering consume microorganisms near the surface of the water. The larvae possess a protection mechanism that lets them move around in an distinctive "S" motion when startled which is why they are referred to as "wigglers" or "wrigglers." The larvae grow out of their exoskeletons as they eat food and develop an entirely new exoskeleton on top of it. Instars refer to the developmental stages which occur between moults. Four instars comprise the stage called larval. The larval stage can last between four and fourteen days dependent on the species and the temperature of the water, as well as the availability of foods.

The stage of pupalization.

Even though there's no food at this stage however, the pupa remains vulnerable to shadows, light as well as other noises. They is required to breathe at the surface of the ocean. Puppye utilize a rolling, or tumbling motion in order to move out of the water and deeper this is the reason they're often described in the term "tumblers." Between 1 1/2 to four days are passed in the period of the pupal stage, until the skin of the pupa splits across the back. This allows the newly formed adult to emerge slowly and get a foothold at the surface of the water.

Adult mosquitoes

In general, the adult male mosquito first emerges and will wait for females near to the breeding area. Because of the high mortality rates, mating occurs immediately after the mosquito's the emergence. Each day, as much as 30% of adults may die. To compensate the high mortality rate females lay numerous eggs that ensure the existence of this species. Male mosquitoes generally live between 6 and 7 days. They only consume nectar from plants; they are not able to consume blood. Females usually live for six weeks, but they may live longer than 5 months, or even longer if they have sufficient food. Females typically need to take an elixir of blood as well as nectars from plants in order to nourish and develop her eggs. They find their victims through the patterns of temperature they produce and trace molecules that they release like carbon dioxide. They are highly vulnerable to several chemicals, such as octenol amino acids, as well as carbon dioxide. A typical female mosquito will travel between 10 and one kilometer, and certain species may travel up to 40 miles before consuming blood. Female mosquitoes be ovipositing (laid) her eggs at the end of every blood meal, completing the entire life cycle. A few species only oviposit one time while others will perform it several times over their life.

Chapter 15: The Mosquito

The insect group that is known as diptera or insects, also known as flies, include mosquitoes. Indeed it is they are the Spanish term used to describe mosquitoes"small fly" is "small fly." The expression "two wings" or "diptera" is a reference to the characteristic which distinguishes flies from the other species of insects. Protoscis of mosquitoes, which is long and tubular, mouthparts designed to sucking liquids. The scales which resemble hairs that cover its body, distinguish it from the other types of insect.

Female or Anophelus mosquitoes

The average lifespan of a female mosquito can be measured in months or weeks. Males usually only need one or two weeks to live. The public is not as familiar with the larval stage of the mosquito. They lay their eggs within areas that been recently full of water. They develop into larvae that resemble worms, and tend to float on the surface they breathe in tubes attached to their tails and eat tiny organisms such as bacteria. In the end, most mosquito larvae need an environment that is organic including leaves, or sewage, in order to serve as a food source for bacteria the mosquito larvae eat.

Incubating larvae from hatchlings can develop to comma-like pupae within one week. The mosquito larvae are often called "wigglers" because they wiggle with ferocity when the environment is disturbed, mosquito pupae are often referred to as "tumblers" because they tumble in the waters. The stage that is called the pupal mosquito is not fed however, the respiratory system of its pupae is comparable to the one of adults and larvae. The pupa usually develops into a mature mosquito within 3 days.

The normal life-cycle of mosquitoes includes a handful of notable differences. The predatory larvae of certain species of mosquito develop into adults who feed on blood Certain larvae of mosquito species consume the larvae of species.

Each female mosquito species will have a preference for the blood type they choose to consume. While some mosquitoes feed off those of reptiles as well as amphibians. Most mosquitoes feast on both mammals and birds. Since blood meals are usually required to lay eggs Female mosquitoes only are stinging. A few types of female mosquitoes as well as the majority of male mosquitoes don't bite. Instead of taking blood for food, they consume nectar as well as other liquids from plants.

Mosquitoes have the ability to locate individuals and species they'd like to attack with a range of signals. They can detect carbon dioxide released by their hosts, at some feet away. Mosquitoes are able to detect body compounds such as lactic acid, which is found in sweat.

The mosquitoes favor certain types of people over other. Someone who is sleeping in a area that has a large number of mosquitoes could wake up by bites. However, people who are close to them might not be bitten. Like how humans react differently to bites caused by insect bites, some sufferers exhibit no evidence that they have been bit while others have significant swelling, itching as well as redness. The severity the severity of an allergic response saliva from mosquitoes varies from individual to person.

A few mosquitoes travel further than 20 miles away from the source of their water which spawned them due to their extensive distance of flight. But, they fly at about 4 miles an hour. In the case of windy days, less mosquitoes can be seen since they usually fly towards the wind in order to find any scents that the host has.

The mosquito is looking for signs of things that are dark when it is close to its target. If it finds the victim, it flew across, lies down, and uses the proboscis to search for blood vessels under the skin. It inspects for wounds and then injects saliva into the wounds. A substance that prevents blood clotting in saliva guarantees the blood circulation is constant and continuously. The saliva of mosquitoes can also be contaminated by viruses, such as the encephalitis-related virus as well as parasites that can cause malaria. That's how the mosquito-borne diseases can be transmitted.

Culex mosquitoes

Culex mosquitoes mostly transmit West Nile virus. Medium-sized Culex mosquito features white stripes across its abdomen and has a brown color. This includes the indoor house moths (C. pipiens as well as C. quinquefasciatus) as well as the more common indigenous species found in the mosquito with western encephalitis (C. Tarsalis). The evenings and sunset, they typically bite. They sleep during the daytime within and around structures and the vegetation.

Culex laid "rafts" of eggs on still waters in a myriad of locations, both artificial and natural including trees, ditches and sewerage systems, waters, trap basins (storm drains) as well as non-chlorinated swimming and wading pool, attractive pools, bird baths buckets, flower pots, empty tires, clogged gutters as well as water-retaining rubbish and other debris. Culex cannot grow when there is water that is moving or that is present for a shorter period of time than. Therefore, all efforts should be made to prevent the accumulation of water in containers or, at minimum, empty containers of water at least once per week.

The distance adult Culex mosquitoes cover to reach maturity isn't too impressive. House mosquitoes may "over-winter" in protected areas such as crawl spaces, sewers as well as basements, in contrast to other mosquitoes which die with the appearance to the first heavy frosts of the fall.

Aedes mosquitoes

Many mosquito species that are bothersome and species that carry diseases can be located in the Aedes mosquito family. There are a variety of mosquito species who prefer eating mammal blood are the inland floodwater mosquito (Aedes Vexans) and the Asian Tiger mosquito (Aedes albopictus) as well as trees hole mosquito (Ochlerotatus triseriatus*). Floodwater mosquitoes lay eggs which allow the larvae to develop in temporary pools, and then eggs to develop into eggs. Container breeders Asian tree holes and tiger mosquitoes lay their eggs in tiny water-filled crevices such as stumps, tree holes wood, logs and even the man-made container like old tires.

Mosquitoes who live in floodwaters that are inland have brownish B-shaped marks around their stomachs. They are particularly unpleasant in low-lying regions including backwaters from rivers, are flooded.

They're usually the first insect to be observed during the spring, and then later after lots of rain. In many cases, there are so many adults emerging at once from the flooded regions that natural barriers like parasites and predators have been overwhelmed.

Contrary to others Aedes insect species in-line floodwater mosquitoes travel for more than 10 kilometers in search of blood meal. They may bite more than other species of Illinois. The majority of them fly towards the end of afternoon and most active at night, however they are able to bite anytime during the day, especially if they are afraid while sleeping in heavily forested and shady areas. It is fortunate that they seldom do, if ever, bring about illnesses within the United States, and they typically die in the fall, when they experience the first snowflake.

White and black insects which bite throughout the day are called Asian Tiger Mosquitoes (see image on the page). They arrived in this nation in the year 1985, and then dispersed throughout a number of states which included Illinois as part of tire shipment. It is not clear what the Asian Tiger mosquito is able to transmit West Nile and

LaCrosse encephalitis to human beings and animals, the Asian tiger mosquito has the potential of sustaining both virus.

The mosquito that bites trees is the principal mosquito vector (carrier) in LaCrosse Encephalitis. The mosquito is silvery white with stripes on the side of the thorax as well as its abdomen, and it is dark-colored. The mosquito that lives in trees, as with the Asian Tiger mosquito, bites throughout the day. They deposit their eggs in tiny containers that the water collects, such as the holes in trees, old tires, buckets, cans and barrels. They are usually found around the woody areas.

The mosquito that lives in the tree hole, Ochlerotatus triseriatus, was previously was known as Aedes triseriatus.

Chapter 16: Mosquito-Borne Encephalitis Diseases

Meningitis as well as viral encephalitis carried by mosquitoes share similar life cycle. They are both associated with different species of birds that are believed to be reservoirs. These species usually don't suffer any severe damage when they are bitten by mosquitoes infected. They are able to create enough virus inside their bodies to cause mosquitoes at least for a brief period. In the manner described above, mosquitoes are able to carry the ability to transmit the virus to different species, which includes birds, horses and even humans. Since they don't generate enough viruses to cause infection in people, mosquitoes, and horses generally are considered "dead-end" hosts. So, the transmission of diseases occurs only between dead-end hosts.

It's hard to know the amount of cases of encephalitis in humans will happen in any particular time. Certain types of encephalitides are believed to be recurring frequently. Health issues of birds that are infected from a large reservoir may be the reason for this. After a short time after getting infected, birds could still be infected with enough virus to aid mosquitoes who bite them carry the disease. Once they have passed that point, they're not an active reservoir for the virus. There are fewer birds around to transfer the disease to mosquitoes as the number of birds that live in an area reach the infective phase. In the end, there are fewer mosquitoes with the virus and less cases of infection.The periodic nature of certain viruses can be significantly affected by the fluctuation in the ratio of infected and. non-infectious bird species in the community. Naturally, there are numerous other variables at play. These include that of the supply of food as well as other resources that have an effect on the amount of the bird population; availability of locations in which mosquito larvae may form, which can have an impact on the amount of mosquito populations. Also, the weather conditions, such as temperatures and rainfall.

West Nile Diseases

There is a West Nile virus has emerged as the apex infection that insects and all other animals closely related to these, including mosquitoes, other flies with bites as well as ticks, vectors (transmit). Birds or mosquitoes that are infected with their own West Nile virus when they arrived in the United States in 1999. There were 884 cases of the virus and 67 deaths from West Nile illness in 2002, Illinois ranked first in the US.

West Nile virus utilizes birds and/or other animals as reservoirs for exist, as do any other virus that causes encephalitis. A majority of mammals as well as birds are immune However, mosquitoes who bit them could eat the virus and transmit the virus to other animals, for instance, humans.

Crows, blue jays horses, squirrels and even humans are one of the species and animals that this virus may affect more than other species and can cause severe illness and the death. But, once infected with the virus, nearly the majority of people have none of the symptoms and have some form of temporary immunity. The elderly and those with weaker immune systems are significantly more likely to develop West Nile fever, a virus that is similar to flu and can last for several weeks or even lead to deadly complications that affect the nervous system such as meningitis and encephalitis.

St. Louis Encephalitis

The virus responsible for St. Louis encephalitis is like West Nile virus and is additionally transmitted through Culex mosquitoes. It has been associated with recurring epidemics among humans. St. Louis encephalitis has been much less prevalent within the United States than West Nile virus. It typically has a limited impact on the south of the nation, specifically in the Mississippi Valley. St. Louis encephalitis has less potential to trigger outbreaks in comparison to West Nile virus. The largest epidemic, first recognized within St. Louis, Missouri and occurred during the mid-late 1970s. Approximately 2000 human cases were recorded. The virus is stored on reserve in the birds.

Eastern and Western Equine Encephalitides

Encephalitis viruses that are closely linked are not often responsible for outbreaks. Eastern Equine Encephalitis is believed to be spread through a variety of distinct species of mosquito, while Western Equine Encephalitis is transmitted through the Culex Tarsalis mosquito, which is also called the western encephalitis mosquito. Because equine encephalitides could be the most dangerous for mortalities among the encephalitides that exist, it's beneficial that they're not more prevalent.

California Encephalitides

Along with producing a mild illness for people, this specific category of encephalitis viruses is distinct from other viruses in the sense that animals, rather than birds, act as reservoirs of the virus.

LaCrosse is considered to be the largest and most widespread form of the California Encephalitis virus that is prevalent in the Midwest. LaCrosse is the predominant strain in the Midwest. LaCrosse virus is distinctive by the fact that it predominantly affects children. Furthermore, since the virus is able to spread between female mosquitoes and the offspring of her, it's not required for mosquitoes to consume an infected person in order to be infected.

LaCrosse-related encephalitis is not usually a cause of the death of a person, but it could result in seizures or other issues related to the nervous system youngsters that may last for many years. The mosquito that bites trees, Ochlerotatus triseriatus is the person who transmits the illness. After eating chipmunks and squirrels and stinging people, the mosquito bites them. The rodents are found in wooded areas, and have been linked to LaCrosse Encephalitis. It is more likely to develop of LaCrosse encephalitis when vehicles and garbage pile in close proximity to woodland places due to the insect larvae of the tree hole develop inside natural cavities and made-up containers. Additionally, adults don't fly too far from their sites for development of larvae.

Chapter 17: Preventing Mosquito Bites

Prevention is one way of getting rid of bites from mosquitoes. But, mosquitoes are still able to bite you even when you're spending your entire mosquito season in the shade. They, just like those in the home can be found getting into buildings and feeding upon occupants, while using cellars, crawlspaces, and cellars to provide quiet areas to rest for winter. The integrity of window or door screens as well as weather stripping is essential in addition to screening and sealing any holes that mosquitoes may use to gain access into the structure such as the areas in the vicinity of vents, utilities lines foundation cracks spaces around doors and windows.

First line of protection against bites from mosquitoes is using repellents. Many products provide a certain amount of protection against mosquito bites. Certain active substances have a higher level of protection. DEET (N,N-diethyl-meta-toluamide) has served as the industry standard for many years. Its products with between 20% and 30 percent DEET provide protection against mosquitoes that can last for a long time in the event of use as indicated in the label. Even though there are products that contain greater DEET concentrations, they usually don't provide much more protection.

Recent research have shown that items containing picaridin, the active ingredient, provide the same degree of protection but do not have the taste or stickiness that is present in DEET-based products. The third ingredient, citrus oil, which is derived from eucalyptus is a plant-derived chemical that also provides security, but not longer than that provided through products containing DEET or picaridin.

If you are planning to apply any repellent for yourself or your child be sure to adhere to the instructions on the package. Application of repellents containing the oil of lemon from eucalyptus on young children isn't recommended.

Managing mosquitoes

Larviciding, or the application of chemical substances for killing mosquito larvae, before they turn into bite-inducing adults has proven to be the most effective method for the control of mosquitoes. In providing advice and funding to local health departments as well as other organizations that conduct larviciding, as well as mosquito surveillance The Illinois Department of Public Health promotes the control of mosquitoes. To be able to anticipate diseases and mosquito outbreaks surveillance entails the collection and identifying of mosquitoes. Also, it involves the concentration of on the areas of concern for control.

Larviciding

The most common method of larviciding is to douse the water in which mosquito larvae develop using pesticides that contain methoprene Bacillus thuringiensis Israelensis or B. the sphaericus bacterium. The Bacillus is ingested by mosquito larvae when they consume. They die when it ingests the bacterial poison which perforates the intestinal tracts. Methoprene-containing larvacide works by interfering with the larva's metamorphosis, preventing it from turning into an adult. The two varieties of larvacide are believed to be appropriate for use in fish-inhabited water due to their lower concentration of toxicity.

To use for private purposes of their property, homeowners are able to purchase these larvicides from hardware and bargain stores, in addition to gardens and lawn centers. They are a great option for situations when water-filled containers, like ones that hold water for horses, or even decorative swimming pools is difficult or undesirable. It is also possible to do this using goldfish (Carassius) as well as the mosquito species (Gambusia). Others larvicides are used to cover the surface of water by thin layers of liquid as a way to stop the larvae from taking oxygen from the air.

Adulticiding

In addition to insecticides to treat the general area of the property of the application Adulticides require certification for mosquito control by the Illinois Department of Agriculture. The application of small droplets of insecticides in ultra-low volume (ULV) treatment by a specialized trucks or aerial machines is the standard method for stopping adult mosquitoes. The mosquito population in a particular area could be significantly affected with this form method of "fogging." Although adulticiding is a broad spectrum treatment which kills mosquitoes as well as beneficial insects, larviciding kills mosquito larvae in a more selective manner. It is also much more expensive than larviciding needs precise product and equipment calibration, timing and use and the right environment conditions to work (generally at night in the evening when mosquitoes are at their peak and temperatures are between 60 F to 85 F with only a little breeze). Larviciding must be utilized alongside adulticiding if the mosquito population is too high in the area or if excessive mosquito-borne viruses pose the public health risk. When the usage of adulticides is considered and mosquito control measures such as taking care to capture mosquitoes and then checking them for diseases such as the West Nile virus can assist to determine the possibility of spread in a particular location. Before the beginning of any treatments it is essential that the general public be informed, and any questions or questions should be answered.

Certain adulticides may also be applied to plants as well as the outdoor areas of buildings and other places which mosquitoes are known to rest and also via fogging. It involves spraying liquid insecticides finely. With regard to the cost as well as environmental impact This kind of treatment is more efficient than fogging and can be more targeted.

By reducing the amount of vegetation that grows surrounding ponds or surrounding your home can help in decreasing the amount of locations that mosquito larvae may develop into adult mosquitoes, and also in which adults are able to rest thus reducing the requirement to spray pesticides on the areas.

Source Reduction

Eliminating the habitat for mosquitoes to develop is perhaps the best way to stop the problem. It is referred to as source reduction. elimination of water sources out of mosquito breeding sites. Ponds, lakes, backwaters and lagoons are able to be cleaned to do this also, and so can the naturally and artificial containers, in order to keep the water out of these. Everyone has a duty to ensure that our property is free of stagnant ponds and poorly maintained swimming pools, trees and empty tires and bird baths, buckets and any other debris areas where water gathers and can be used as a breeding ground for mosquitoes.

What isn't working

Advertisers often make numerous statements about their products that claim for repelling mosquitoes. If they are used in a proper manner, the items mentioned below have proven to work. Here are a few options products that provide little or none protection against mosquitoes.

bats and martins in purple

electrocuting equipment to cut insects

electronic and ultrasonic devices

pseudo-"mosquito plants"

Vitamin or other dietary supplements

Many tools to capture mosquitoes are being developed in recent times. A lot of mosquito repellents do not work. Some might be effective in catching large quantities of mosquitoes. However, traps are expensive as there's no evidence that their use reduces the chance of contracting a illness transmitted by mosquitoes. The most effective methods to prevent bites from mosquitoes are the reduction of sources, application of pesticides as well as the application of repellents for mosquitoes.

Chapter 18: Malaria

Malaria continues to kill and cause ill health in a vast scale particularly among vulnerable populations, babies and women who are pregnant in areas of tropical. In Africa the disease causes over one million deaths per year. And in Nigeria the rates of infection is deemed to be insidious, with greater than 75 percent of kids with a age range of between 5 and 9 years of age being affected.

Antimalarial medications have been utilized in a variety of ways to stop or treat malaria within the populations living in malaria-prone areas for more than two decades. The alarming pace at which this parasite, specifically Plasmodium falciparium has been able to evolve resistance to the currently widely used drugs to treat malaria and makes it necessary to look for more advanced, more efficient therapeutic methods.

The need for this has been highlighted in the latest suggestion of artemisinin (a plant-derived product) combined therapies based on plant products by the World Health Organisation (WHO). Artemisinin is a plant product that comes from Artemisia annua, as well as quinine, derived in Cinchona species, are both proven instances of substances that are derived from plants and have anti-malarial properties.

What exactly is malaria?

The Malaria virus is believed to be an infection due to a parasite Plasmodium that infects the red blood cells. Malaria is characterised by a series of fever, chills sweating and pain. The evidence from the past suggests that the spread of malaria to humans has been evident since the dawn of time. The term "mal 'aria" (meaning "bad air" in Italian) was first coined to describe the disease in English around 1740, by H. Walpole when describing the illness. The term was later merged into "malaria" in the 20th century. A.C. Laveran, in 1880, was the first researcher to discover the blood parasites that cause malaria in humans. In 1889, Dr.

Ronald Ross a British army surgeon stationed in India found that mosquitoes carried malaria. According to Ross, out there are four kinds that are malaria-related, the more dangerous kind of malaria is Plasmodium falciparum malaria. It is life-threatening. Three other types that are malaria (P. Vivax, P. malariae, and P. ovale) tend to be less dangerous and don't pose any risk to your life.

What is the method of transmission for malaria?

The researchers said that malaria can be transmissible to humans when the mosquito that is infected bites someone and injects malaria-causing parasites (sporozoites) into the bloodstream. Sporozoites move through bloodstream and into the liver. They maturing, and then affect red blood cells of the human. When red blood cells are infected it is possible for the parasites to appear when a mosquito consumes the blood of someone who is infected and then ingests the human blood vessels that contain the parasites. After that, the parasites enter to the Anopheles mosquito's stomach. They eventually infiltrate the salivary glands of mosquitoes. In the event that Anopheles mosquitos bite a human being, these sporozoites finish their Plasmodium development cycle. P. ovale as well as P. Vizax may make the cycle more complicated in the form of dormant stage (hypnozoites) which may not be developed for several weeks or years.

Does Mosquito Cause Malaria?

The globe has embraced this tale and discovered, hook, line and sinker that malaria due to Anopheles mosquito. According to the malaria theory, that when an Anopheles mosquito bites an individual and injects malaria-causing parasites into blood after which the parasites develop which eventually causes infection of red blood cells of the human. In red blood cells there is a recurrence of the parasites after a mosquito consumes the blood of an affected human, and then bites someone else, the parasite spreads. You will be interested to know that a mosquito bites people once before dying. The mosquito that is sucks blood can continue to suck, thus why would mosquito become an agent for transmission?

This is because the goal of exploration is to provide a solutions to a problem that is already in place The root of a problem discovered is the problem that is half-solved. Let's find out if the discoveries brought relief to the threat of malaria and mosquitoes. the evidence from history suggests that malaria has been a major cause of infection for humans.

since the dawn of time. in 1740, a whopping two decades before, malaria was identified after H. Walpole, equally in 1880, Alphonse. Laveran identified the blood parasites that cause malaria in 1889. In the following year, Sir Ronald Ross a British army surgeon who was stationed in India observed that mosquitoes transmit malaria. From that time, the world has been fighting to eliminate malaria and mosquitoes and malaria, however nothing has worked. It is believed that the World Health Organization and other health organizations of other countries have spent and continue to spend billions of dollars to fight mosquitoes and malaria. The Nigerian government Nigeria invested N17 million during 2009/2010 in fighting malaria and mosquitoes. Markets are brimming with various mosquito-treated nests, mosquito repellents mosquito repellents, mosquito coils and more.

Listen carefully, and learn what the experts say, that mosquito which has been said to be the cause of malaria can't be eliminated. Can man fight God? Mosquito is one kinds of insects that were designed by God with a specific purpose, that no human being can fully eradicate any creation of God. (We will discuss why mosquitos exist as well as other insect species in a later issue)

It was said that water stagnation, unclean environments and poverty are the primary cause for malaria and other ailments, but I do not agree (in principle) due to the wealth and rich individuals living in pest control environment, mansions sporting screens all over the dwelling, drinking bore hole treated water as well as other drinking water bottles, 24/7 automobiles and air-conditioned homes as well suffer from the effects of malaria. The fact is that mosquitoes don't even know what they taste like on their skin. But they continue to suffer from the malaria-related illness and are able to spend a significant amount of money on local doctors to treat them. Don't confuse me. I'm not an advocate to a dirty planet since I'm a proponent for a clean and healthy environment. I am a living and breathing example of it. But that doesn't guarantee the absence of malaria.

A few days ago, I went with an acquaintance to the offices that of a multi-millionaire from Kaduna city in Kaduna state Nigeria to have a discussion about business during which his cell phone rang. The person answering the call seemed to be sympathizing with him in being admitted to hospital for malaria as well as the typhoid. The millionaire questioned why he's currently suffering from malaria as well as typhoid, based on the fact the only water he drinks is treated borehole water other than treated boreholes and water that is bottled.

Friends, the entire issue has become clearer drinking water treated is certainly not a guarantee to not be afflicted with typhoid or malaria because the water treated is saturated with a recognized and deadly immune suppressants known as chlorine. Chlorine is the byproduct from nuclear waste. As an aforementioned poison, it gradually destroys organs like kidneys and liver, and degrades the immune system and the body's capacity to recognize and eliminate toxic substances. It is possible that you don't know this since you've been sanitized and rehydrated and instructed to drink treated water in order to avoid the water-borne illnesses.

If you're interested, the last time I was there, my brother-in-law as well as his Lebanese acquaintance received an agreement with Kaduna the state-owned water board of Nigeria to provide chemical products for water treatment, with chlorine as one. After they received the chemicals comprising chlorine, they set up the chemical outside since it is in cylinders. However, the next day a potentially dangerous incident occurred. The grasses surrounding where they had parked their chlorine cylinders had died and withered and the other creatures that walked around (dogs as well as goats) were also killed. They managed to locate the leaky the cylinder and towing it by a car and and dropped it in the river and it neutralized the effect and killed fish that were in the water where the cylinder was dropped. If you are treating your water with chlorine, or it's byproducts, no regardless of the brand name such as water protector, water shield or any other, it kills every good mineral element within the water. It will leave empty, however it makes the water a an ineffective killer that is ready to weaken body organs. People who drink water treated will first be sick on days when they consume regular water as the chlorine in water has weakened the immune system, which helps the body protect itself from and fight infections.

Top water treatment

The best method treatment for your water purchase filters and connect them with the water source that is your supply. I'm talking about the pipe of water that runs to your kitchen, or into your storage tank. Secondly, you could purchase table top filters. Maybe you can't afford this but if you can do it yourself, add water to your storage containers and let the water get settled over the night, or for a few hours. You will then are drinking healthy and safe water.

The Real Causes of Malaria

The main cause of malaria is poor diet, that causes low immune which results in the body not being able to defend itself. body to protect itself. Plasmodium (now known as malaria parasite) originates from Plasma as a human blood components. When the body is functioning normally plasma, which is a clear yellow fluid, is a conduit for blood flow to various cells within the body. If there's an imbalance within the body's mechanism caused by poor diet and the accumulation of toxins organs and body features are likely to alter their appearance and forms, and cells begin dying due to a lack of blood in the plasma. If this occurs and a tests for blood are conducted sure, the results will reveal dead cells that are seeking methods of getting out of the body. and this is referred to as malaria parasite. Where is the malaria parasite coming from? External or internal? Do I dare to tell to you that the malaria virus is an inside illness which is not a problem externally, and therefore the mosquito cannot be responsible.

Fresh, healthy and fresh nutrition promotes healthy well-being (strong and active immune system) and junk, processed and processed foods suppress the immune system, paving ways for clogging (constipation) as well as the deterioration of body systems, leading to illness and illness. Medical experts and scientists have generally agreed that the primary reason for illness is toxemia (constipation) an obstruction of the whole organ system that is the pipe of our body. In this case, toxins are released into the bloodstream because of putrefaction. Daniel and his men consumed fresh, healthy food and they lived longer and were more knowledgeable than other men who ate the royal diet (junk artificial, processed and cooked foods) Daniel 1:8, 12 13:15, 8. 8"But Daniel was determined not to contaminate himself through eating food or the wine provided to them by the King. He questioned the chief of staff permission to consume the forbidden food items. ...Vs12 We must be tested for ten days following eating a balanced diet consisting of fruits and vegetables, as well as drinking water. Daniel said. Vs. 13 At the conclusion of the 10 days, look at the way we appear compared to those young men have been eating the food provided by the king. Verse. 15 At conclusion of the ten-day period, Daniel and three of his friends were healthier and had better nutrition as compared to the other young people who were eating food provided by the King". (New Living Bible)

If you are eating unacceptably foods of the king? You are creating the conditions for health problems. If a blood test reveals it is found that there are malaria parasites (Plasmodium falciparum) or Salmonella when it comes to Typhoid, good for you! There is no reason to be concerned, but rather it's a signal that their body is weakened due to toxicemia. Therefore, the body demands cleansing as well as the ingestion of appropriate foods to strengthen your immune system (body defence). If the body is not functioning because of degeneration in organs sure the body will show it in the blood. Why is that? The life of flesh is contained in blood', the Bible declared in Leviticus 17:11-14. The secret of living and health lies in blood. This is why any illness can be identified through bloodstream, e.g. diabetics, typhoid, malaria, HIV/AIDS, etc. It will all be gone once this mystery is comprehended. Organs that are healthy produce pure and clean blood (good health) and weaker organs create impure and polluted blood (sickness). When blood is in the state that is an alkaline state (clean clean and clear) there is no pathogen that can reside it, however when the blood is acidic (impure) the body's systems can be prone to dysfunction. It's not some kind of theoretical article on health but an actual fact.

Prior to my study of nutrition and nutrition, recalcitrant (re-occurring) malaria used to be an everyday occurrence each month. However, in 2002 and up to the present, I am in a malaria-free environment, which includes my family members. From three months until

complete my program and return to Nigeria In September 2004, specifically, my wife informed me by email that my daughter (she was just nine at the time) had stubborn malaria and typhoid that has resisted every prescription for medical. When I returned in December of 2004, she was in a state of anemia and looked pale. instantly I took action and put the girl onto honeygal (honey and vinegar) as well as other live food and within a few days, she was fully recovered and to date she has never been afflicted by malaria. Thanks to the mercy of God others have also been taking advantage of this information and are now free from the dreadful threat of malaria. The identical.

Chapter 19: Factors Which Reduce Our Immune System

The body's capability to defend its body from attack by inflicting malaria parasites, viruses, fungi, bacteria cancer and so on is influenced due to a variety of causes. Each of us has had sudden cold-like symptoms that occurs following the stress of a life event like a long period of joy, divorce and loss of job and so on. The stress of these events may reduce our immunity and put us at risk of numerous ailments. Insufficient nutrition, poor diet as well as stress and emotional stress, poisons from the environment and abuse of medications or exercise routines are all factors that contribute to the weakness of the immune system to guard and defend us. The good news is that our bodies can be extremely regenerative, and our own body of immune cells can be boosted in a matter of weeks just by improving the nutrition we consume. When we eat the correct kinds of foods that are immune-specific and reducing stress levels, the balance of our emotions and exercising regularly can help to boost the weakening immune system.

Good Food

Quality and good food items are not measured by cost or country of origin (in instances of import products) rather by the quality of the enzymes you get from the food you eat. A lot of people believe that buying and eating costly canned foods and beverages laced with all sorts of additives can keep you well, however I can tell you that this is not true. People who eat synthetic and technology-based food, develop the technological illnesses known as big-man illness (diabetics as well as hypertension as well as impotency, fainting and other symptoms). If the quality of life depends on how much the food we consume costs and the rich can never be sick.

Food that is healthy includes at least 50% of fresh, natural food (fruits as well as vegetables) as well as 50 percent cooked food.

What is Food?

Food is food that you should consume. According to science the word "food" refers to either a solid or liquid that performs any vital functions for the human body. In order to keep your body operating optimally, it is essential to eat to grow and also for bodily activities. It is also required to provide energy, construct and maintain tissues in the body and regulate bodily processes. The proper nutrition is evident the well-built body.

Nutrition

The study of nutrition is the way that our body gets nourished. The research of nutrition is focused on the structure of the food and how it serves to keep tissues of the body in good health. The diverse parts of organs and tissues remain in a constant state of flux. When you are a child, there is fast growth of all cells in the body. When you are an adult, your tissues are continuously repaired and preserved. Though changes are happening throughout the body all the moment, it's a regular process and process of the body continues with a regular pace. The process of change in chemical which occurs in living cells, which results in the creation of new tissues, the breakdown of tissues that have been damaged and the production of energy, is known as metabolism.

A nutritious diet is required to support all the changes that occur within the cells that are developing.

The science of food has classified it into four groups, which include proteins, carbohydrate as well as fats and vitamins (other foods mentioned earlier require vitamins in order to function. How much vitamins are you taking at each meal is a significant factor to maintain your well-being. It is possible to get more information about food combinations at the time you get me to talk one-on-one.

Take note of your food choices and be aware that it can affect the life of your loved ones. Many people have allergies directly related to the food they consume or consume. Allergies are an unintentional negative reaction to a chemical that can affect one person however, not everyone. Allergies can come in many shapes and sizes and can be accompanied by a variety of signs and they can cause in the form of just about everything. If you suffer from allergies or are frequently feeling tired, fatigued and depressed for living, it could be beneficial to take a serious and close review of your current food habits. A lot of allergies can be caused by foodstuffs that contain colourings, food additives and preservatives as well as taste enhancers such as monosodium glutamate (MSG). Monosodium glutamate (MSG) is present within Maggi cubes Royco cubes Knorr cubes Ajinomoto and many more. Researchers in the field of nutrition have been involved about foods that cause strange reactions for the past 25 years. The majority of food products consumed today may have no value or be detrimental to your health. If they're useless then they're nothing anything more than waste of your energy, time as well as money. If they're dangerous then they shouldn't be a part of your food regimen at all. These types of foods can cause issues for health when you go between sickness and feeling good. Ineffective and unhealthy foods can hinder your body's capacity to perform optimally and could hinder your desire to achieve total wellbeing.

Salt

The regular consumption of table salt disrupts the balance of sodium and potassium which can cause health issues to occur. These include hypertension as well as premenstrual stress, swelling of ankles, feet, and kidney issues. Reduced sodium intake will limit the potential for these problems. In addition you could want to increase the amount of potassium, such things as oranges, bananas as well as whole grains. Plantains are also a good source of potassium.

Sugar

A high intake of refined sugar may cause lasting issues over the long term. Consuming a diet that is laden with sweets soft drinks, caffeine-sweetened beverages and teas harms your health and sets the base for obesity, hypoglycemia as well as asthma, arthritis, circulation and heart condition, tooth decay, and a variety of behavioral problems. Sugar deprives you of the vital vitamin C that is part of the family of B-complexes. It causes an imbalance of the ratio of calcium and phosphorus that is crucial for the overall health of your bones and teeth.

Alcohol

For some, alcohol may be enjoyable as an occasional drink for others, while to some may consider it a daily ritual. If it's a casual or a regular occasion, drinking alcohol is known to cause liver diseases or circulatory and heart diseases and can cause severe temperament and personality shifts. The consumption of alcohol can result in obesity. It causes complications to all disorders or illnesses that one might have.

Fat

A diet high in fat, especially that is comprised of mainly saturated fats such as margarine, palm oil, butter, etc. puts a lot of stress on the body. Palm oil is great for your eyes due to its vitamin A. But what's the its negative impact on the heart as it is a source of saturated fat (That's why it smokes during cooking) saturated fat can slow digestion and also the absorption of vital nutrients, and eventually can result in liver, circulatory and cardiac illnesses. To reduce your intake of fats, consume mainly low-fats with no saturated content (like groundnut oil in its original form or cotton seed oil olive oil and mustard oil) Reduce the intake of the animal fat (red meat, and butter) out of your diet in order to avoid cholesterol accumulation within your arteries.

Tea and Coffee

A cup of coffee on occasion or tea can be rejuvenating and relaxing, however the continuous consumption of both beverages could cause addiction and damage your well-being. Coffee and tea contain caffeine which is a chemical that can be detrimental on the nervous system and mucous membranes, lining of the stomach and the intestine. Gastritis-related disorders and indigestion, as well as hypertension as well as peptic ulcers can take away vitamin B. These are the nutrients needed to treat the symptoms. You can try decaffeinated or tea in the event that you are unable to eliminate these beverages completely from your life. The consumption of coffee and tea isn't necessary; you can continue to be enjoyable with the need for them. We Africans because from "long-throat" go ahead to drink them even though our climate does not require an ongoing heating process because of cold. Since we have seen the people of the white race eating them fast, we began to incorporate both coffee and tea in our daily diet.

Chemical Food Additives, Drugs, Solvents, Pesticides, Herbicides, Dyes, Artificial Sweeteners, Food Colouring

These can all find ways into your body and start to harm the health of your body. There are many food additives that dyes, and preservatives are harmful or natural, however it is crucial to understand which products you purchase and eat contains chemical compounds and what the chemicals contain. Recently, many individuals have removed specific food additives from their diets, and observed that such as the symptoms of respiratory, skin or nerve ailments disappeared. If you think your health issues are result of your food choices take a look at the possibility that additives are an element in the problem. Details about the most widely utilized food additives is easily accessible. In the developed world the food industry is obliged to declare the ingredients in their products on their label. Certain foods have natural colours however some contain dyes or artificial colouring. Some of these chemicals that create colour by reflecting light, are energy molecules that can interact with and damaging deoxyribonucleic acids (DNA) cells. They are the genetic cells which contain data

164

regarding how your body functions. Anything that causes damage to deoxyribonucleic Acid (DNA) may harm the immune system, increase ageing and trigger diseases such like cancer, and various other chronic illnesses. The majority of food dyes made from synthetic substances believed to be safe become carcinogenic. Food scientists strongly recommend consumers to stay clear of foods that contain artificial colors. They're the ones which cause all sorts of illness.

Food Preservatives

Beware of that chemical preservative if it has Alum (an Aluminum compound) and Nitrites, etc. Some synthetic preservatives such as they are not healthy. Alum, an aluminum-based ingredient used in a variety of kinds of pickles, and also to improve crispness in other meals (Chips, Cheese Bud) is not a good fit in our health and can be detrimental for you. Baking powders may have aluminum in it. Nitrites that are added to various cured meats, aren't in themselves cancer-causing, but they are able to interact with proteins break down products within the digestive tract and result in carcinogenic compounds known as Ni-Rosamines. Recently NAFDAC, the Nigerian Agency responsible for food and drug regulation, National Agency for Food Drug and Administrative Control (NAFDAC) found a toxic Bromate, a substance that is used to bake bread is carcinogenic, and is likely to cause cancer.

If you are eating food with nitrites like sausages, hot dogs etc make sure you take a dose of vitamin C alongside. It can help neutralize the harmful substances.

Chapter 20: Things You Should Know About Malaria Attack

If scientists as well as different International and regional health organizations which believe the malaria epidemic is caused by mosquitoes are unable to keep malaria and mosquitoes in check and malaria, then it isn't an illness, but a symptom that is a condition of the body, which demands the self-examination of oneself and changes in the way of life. If there's one group in God's creations which should be dying in a masse of complex malaria-related illness, it's animals since they're regularly being bitten by mosquitoes. Discover why they thrive despite bites from mosquitoes even more given that malaria has been found to have a tendency to resist the available anti-malaria drugs. What are our options?

Remedy/Practical Tips

I've always believed there are two sides of every illness that is the pure and spiritual physical illness. Any person who is suffering from spiritual or physical illness will eventually develop exhibit symptoms that point towards one or more of the kinds of illnesses. Don't let yourself die before you're ready, research the place where you fall If you are unable to figure it out, I'd love to be able to help.

Spiritual Remedy

In the James chapter 5:13-15. James chapter 5:13-15"

Jam 5:13. Are any one of you suffering? let him pray. Does he seem happy? let him sing psalms.

Jam 5:14. Are there any one of you sick? Let him ask the pastors and elders of the church and then let

Then they pray over them, anointing them with oil, in honor of God:

5:15 in Jam, and a prayer of faith can heal the sick and God will bring him back up. And should he be guilty of wrongs, they will be forgiven"

That means that each demonic illness is a result of a prayers for delivery. Please follow the remedy that applies to your faith, however I recommend both options, both spiritual prayers of deliverance as well as the therapeutic use of natural remedies.

Clean Environment

Cleanliness is the next to godliness. I believe that the cleanliness of the soul, spirit and body as well as the environment is heaven. In heaven, there's nothing but health. Cockroaches, mosquitoes and flies are the God-given agents that ensure a the cleanliness of our environment. In any setting where they can be seen and their surroundings, you must pay attention. A clean environment coupled with fresh, healthy food sources is healthy.

Natural and therapeutic remedy

The typhoid and malaria diseases are among the most deadly illnesses in Africa Today, people are not killed by malaria parasites but instead due to the strong anti-malaria chemical hard drugs. Prior to killing the malaria parasite and typhoid, they've already destroyed the kidney, liver and spleen using chemically-based drugs. These drugs have wiped out millions of people and helped a few.

For a life free from malaria, you need to cleanse the body. It is the process of eliminating the toxins (impurities) out of the body. It is essential to follow a trained guide for this. If you combine Vitamin A, B and and C and immune booster is a way to help you get malaria to be eliminated. Utilize natural sources of vitamin C, such as the pawpawpaw, which is half-ripe and unripe, or Lime, leaf as well as pineapple and lemongrass. The combination of these will help to flush out any malaria that may be present and help protect against the recurrence.

Method One: Materials include 15 slices of lime five slices of lemon 1 half or unripe, unripe and mature pawpaw or leaves and lemon grass. Make sure to wash everything with clear water. Cut the lemon and lime into two pieces, and then chop the pineapple and pawpaw in cubes (If you're using leaves from pawpaws, you can add three pieces) lemon grass include 3 tablespoons (handful or whatever amount that your palm can handle). Pour all of it into an unclean pot and add 3 liters of water (2 large swan bottles equals 3 Liters) and boil it for 30 mins, then allow the mixture to cool.

to cool. Drinking: Half glass/stainless cups twice daily (Before breakfast, and then 30 minutes following dinner). You shouldn't use sugar in this drink, however you could add pure honey for sweetness or take it as is. Beware: It could be too energetic in patients with ulcers. Instead, follow the method below.

Method 2: Grind or squeeze two leaves of pawpaw using 4 glasses of water, then the sieve. Dosage: 1 glass 3 times daily until symptom clears.

Method 3 four: 4 pawpaws with yellow leaves and 30 bitter leaf, squeeze them all into water. (6 Liters of water = 4 large swan water bottles, for measuring. One SWAN bottle measures 1.5 Liters). Dosage: 3 glasses every day over 10 consecutive days.

Hello, the recommendation above isn't exactly scientific or current, but it's the best mixture of minerals and vitamins present in our food fruit and vegetables which we consume are body cleanser in addition to infection fighters/defenders as well as healers. Sincerely, Gods divine providence has allowed me to gain knowledge about nutrition to assist numerous people suffering from terminal or chronic malaria or typhoid heal, and so there is a way to live a life free of the dreadful symptoms of malaria and the typhoid. Get in touch with us to receive further advice.

Chapter 21: Malaria

Malaria is an insect-borne disease that can affect humans as well as species of animals. The symptoms of malaria typically consist of fatigue, fever headaches, vomiting and nausea. If it is severe the disease can cause convulsions, jaundice, deaths, or comas. The symptoms typically manifest ten to 15 days after having been bitten by an infected bug. If treated improperly the patient may suffer repeated episodes of the disease weeks later. If a patient has been through a recent disease, recurrences typically cause less symptoms. The partial resistance decreases with time in the absence of ongoing contact with malaria.

Malaria is triggered by single-celled bacterial strains belonging to the Plasmodium group.

It's spread only through bites from affected Anopheles mosquitoes.

The bite of a mosquito transmits parasites that are present in the saliva of the insect into the blood of a person.

The parasites move into the liver, in which they multiply and grow. Five types of Plasmodium could infect and transmitted by human beings. Most deaths result from P. falciparum. However, P. Vivax, P. ovale, and P. malariae can cause milder forms of malaria. The kind of P. knowslesi rarely causes illness in humans. It is usually diagnosed through studying blood microscopically using blood film, or with antigen-based quick diagnostic tests. Techniques that use an enzyme called polymerase chain reaction detect the DNA of parasites have been created, but do not typically find use in areas that have malaria endemic areas due to the cost and the complexity.

The chance of contracting illness can be decreased by stopping bites from mosquitoes through the use of mosquito nets, insect repellents as well as using techniques for controlling mosquitoes including spraying pesticides, and taking out the standing water. A variety of treatment options are offered to avoid malaria in travelers to areas where malaria spread of the disease is high. Occasional doses of the combination drug sulfadoxine/pyrimethamine are indicated in babies and after the first trimester of pregnancy in locations with a high prevalence of malaria. In 2020, there's a vaccine which has been shown to decrease the risk of contracting malaria by around 40% among children from Africa. Another pre-print study of a vaccination showed 77% effectiveness of the vaccine but this research is not yet undergoing an independent peer review. Needs updating develop more effective vaccines continue. The most common treatment for malaria is an amalgamation of antimalarial medicines that have artemisinin. The second medicine may be either mefloquine, lumefantrine, or sulfadoxine/pyrimethamine. Quinine, when combined with doxycycline may be used if artemisinin unavailable. It is recommended that when the disease is common, malaria be tested for if it is possible before beginning treatment due to the concern of increasing resistance to drugs. Resistance among the parasites has evolved to numerous antimalarial drugs; for example, chloroquine-resistant P. falciparum has spread to most malarial regions, and artemisinin resistance has become a concern in certain parts of Southeast Asia.

The condition is prevalent in the optical environment that occurs across the center of the equator.

It covers the majority of Africa sub-Saharan, Asia, and Latin America.

In the year 2000, the number of instances of malaria in the world, which resulted in the expected death of 627,000. The majority of instances and deaths were in sub-Saharan African. It is often linked to poor living conditions and has a significant negative impact on the growth of economics. In Africa, it's predicted to cost the country 12 billion dollars a year due to increased healthcare costs as well as a lower capacity to work and negative effects on tourism.

Dengue

Dengue disease is tropical infection transmitted by mosquitoes that is caused by dengue viruses. The signs typically manifest after three or fourteen days an infection. They can include high temperature nausea, headache joint and muscular pain along with a noticeable irritation to the skin and a rash. It usually takes between two and seven days. A small percentage of patients, it becomes more serious dengue hemorrhagic disease, resulting in bleeding and low blood platelets as well as bleeding of blood plasma, or in dengue shock syndrome which is characterized by a dangerously lower blood pressure can result.

Dengue is transmitted by a variety of varieties of female mosquitoes from the Aedes Genus, most notably Aedes aegypti. It has five different types of dengue and one of them generally confers permanent immunity for the particular type of virus, however it provides only brief protection for other types.

In the event of an recurrence, infection of another type can lead to severe negative consequences. Numerous tests are readily available to confirm diagnosis, including the detection of antibodies against the virus or DNA.

Dengue fever vaccine has been approved and is widely available in a variety of countries.

Since 2018, vaccination can only be recommended to people who are previously infected or live within areas where there is an increased risk of infections before the age of nine. Another method of preventing it is restricting the habitat of mosquitoes and the exposure to bites. The method is eliminating or securing standing water, as well as wear clothes that cover the bulk parts of the body. Treatment for dengue acute is supportive. It involves delivering liquid either through oral or intravenously to treat moderate or severe disease. In more serious cases the need for a blood transfusion could be required.

Chapter 22: Chikungunya

Chikungunya is a condition that is caused by Chikungunya virus (CHIKV). The symptoms include joint pain and fever. They typically manifest between two and 12 days following exposure.The symptoms can be described as joint pains and fever. Additional symptoms include headaches or muscle pain, joint swelling and itchy rash. The symptoms usually resolve within one week, but occasionally joint pain could persist for years or months. The chance of dying is approximately 1 in 1,000. Younger, older or those who have additional health issues are more at risk for grave illness.

The virus can be spread among people through two varieties of mosquitoes: Aedes albopictus and Aedes the aegypti.

They are most likely to bite during morning. It is possible for the virus to infect many animals, including rodents and birds. It is diagnosed by analyzing the blood samples for virus DNA or antibodies that recognize the virus. It is possible to mistake the symptoms as the symptoms of dengue fever or Zika fever. Most individuals become immune to one virus.

The most effective method of prevention is total mosquito control as well as prevention of bites within areas that are prone to the illness. It can be achieved through limiting mosquito entry to water as well as the recourse to insect repellents as well as mosquito nets. The recommended treatments include rest, liquids, and medication for treating fever and joint pain.

Although the majority of cases occur mostly in Africa and Asia there have been outbreaks documented across Europe as well as the Americas from the early 2000s. More than a million cases were suspected to have occurred. It was a problem in Florida across the continent of United States but as of 2016 there was none of the locally sourced instances. The illness was first discovered by the government of Tanzania. The word comes originated from the Kimakonde dialect and translates as "to become contorted".

Yellow fever

The yellow fever virus is common viral illness with a typical duration of. Most often, the symptoms can include chills, fever nausea, chills, muscles pains, nausea - especially in the back as well as headaches. The symptoms usually improve after five days. About 15% of cases after a few days after improvement, the fever will come again, abdominal pain develops as well as liver damage starts creating the skin to turn yellow. When this happens then the possibility of a kidney infection or bleeding increases.

The cause of the disease is Yellow fever. It is transmitted through bites of the affected mosquito. This virus only affects people, some primates and a variety of different mosquitoes. In urban areas, it's mostly spread through Aedes the aegypti species of mosquito that is found in the subtropics and tropics. It's an RNA virus belonging to the family of Flavivirus. It is possible for the disease to distinguish from other ailments, particularly at the beginning of its course. In order to determine if a patient is suffering from the testing of blood samples using polymerase chain reactions is needed.

A reliable and secure treatment for yellow fever is in place in some countries, while others need vaccinations for visitors. Other measures to stop disease include the reduction of the number of mosquitoes transmitting the virus. In the areas where yellow fever is prevalent, the early detection of the disease and vaccination of large portions of the population is essential to avoid cases. When a person becomes infected the treatment is usually symptomatic. the treatment is not specific enough against the disease. It is possible to die in as much as 50% of people who contract an illness that is severe.

More than a billion people reside in a region that is where the illness is prevalent. The majority of cases are in areas that are tropical, such as those continents South America and Africa, however, it is not so prevalent in Asia. In the past few years there has been an increase in the incidence of yellow fever have increased. It is thought to be because fewer people are susceptible, a greater number of residents living in cities and moving around frequently and the change in climate, which has grown to increase the mosquito breeding grounds.

The disease began in Africa before spreading into the Americas beginning in the 15th century, primarily due to the European trade in slaves Africans who were from Sub-Saharan Africa. From the 17th century onward numerous major outbreaks of this disease have been observed throughout regions like the Americas, Africa, and Europe.

www.ingramcontent.com/pod-product-compliance
Lightning Source LLC
Chambersburg PA
CBHW051727020426
42333CB00014B/1186